T0173466

Is Medicine
Still Good
For Us?

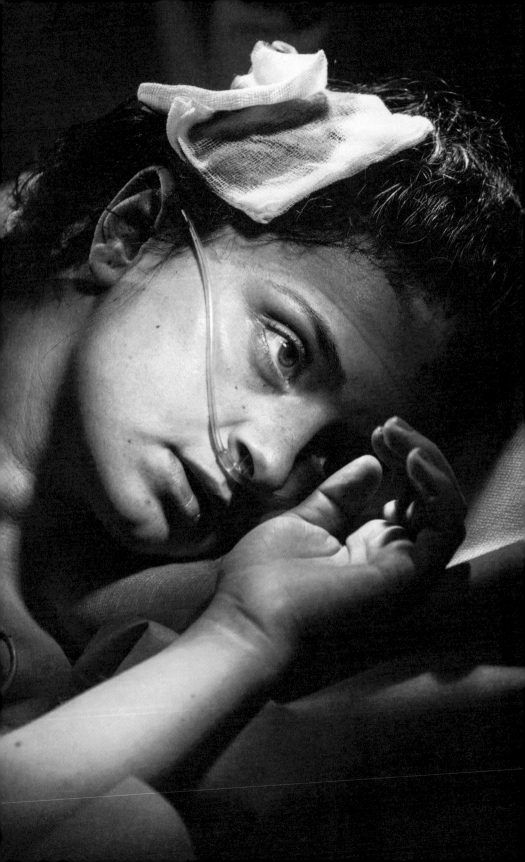

The Big Idea

Julian Sheather

Is Medicine Still Good For Us?

A primer for the 21st century

Over 160 illustrations

Thames & Hudson

General Editor:
Matthew Taylor

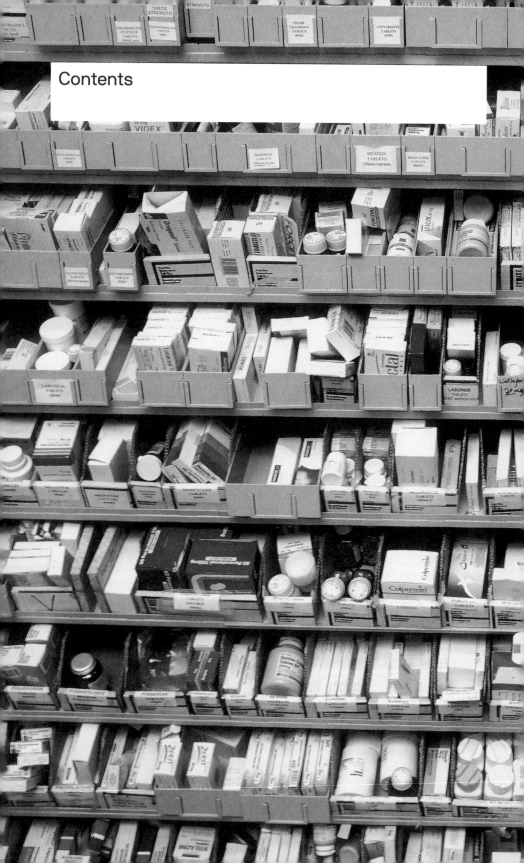

Contents

Introduction   6

1. The Development of Medicine   18

2. How Effective is Medicine?   50

3. The Medicalization of Living and Dying   74

4. Why Modern Medicine Needs to Change   100

Conclusion   128

Further Reading   136

Picture Credits   138

Index   140

Acknowledgments   144

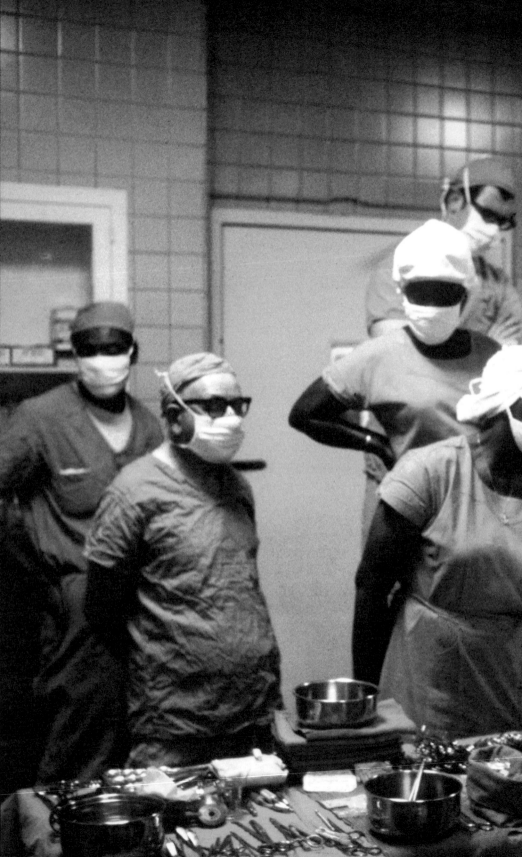

Introduction

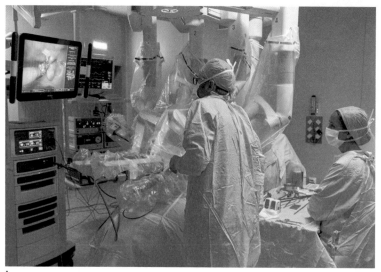

A   Medicine is technologically brilliant – such as this prostate surgery using a Da Vinci surgical robot – but questions remain about both the sustainability of its costs and its cost-effectiveness.

B   Warning signs alert hospital staff and visitors to wash their hands. It is important for visitors to be as vigilant as staff to minimize the spread of nosocomial infections.

A

Western medicine is unparalleled in its global reach and power.

This is linked to Western political and economic hegemony – medicine travelled alongside empire; the biggest (Western) medical companies span the globe – but is also a result of its phenomenal success. Western medicine eradicated polio and performed the first heart transplant. It gave us antibiotics, vaccination and genetic therapy. It has contributed to a stunning increase in life expectancy. Seldom a week passes without media reports of extraordinary breakthroughs. At its best, it is the most humane of our practices, meshing science with clinical judgment and compassionate care to promote our personal flourishing. There is also prestige in the shining institutions of Western healing, the state-of-the-art hospitals, which makes them high points of economic development.

In the decades after World War II, people in the West came largely to believe that, cradle to grave, most of their major health needs would be met. Although there were always tensions and challenges, there was a widespread belief in the progressive overcoming of major threats to health, and, if we did get ill, that our health systems would provide. They would cure where they could and palliate where they could not.

But this consensus is under threat. Transfixed by Western medicine's technological brilliance, its near-miraculous achievements, we have been slow to notice the accumulating downside. Costs and expectations are rising, in some places stratospherically – the USA spends close to 20% of its GDP on health care, for much less than universal coverage – while health returns are shrinking. As expectations increase, so too does awareness of medical risk. Medicine has side effects. Nosocomial infections, adverse reactions, post-operative complications, a range of iatrogenic harms – all the ordinary risks of high-tech medicine sit in the balance sheet alongside the blessings. There are also other disturbing trends.

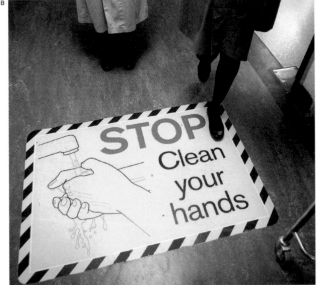

B

Nosocomial Hospital acquired. From the Greek *nosus* (disease) and *komeion* (to take care of). Often refers to infections acquired by patients during their stay in hospital.

Iatrogenic Brought about by the doctor. From the Greek *iatros* (physician) and *genic* (caused or brought about by). Refers to any illness or disease brought about by medical treatment. Iatrogenic illness is a key risk factor for medical treatment.

Modern medicine is inconceivable without antibiotics, but immunity is surging through overuse.

In the USA, dependence on prescription opioids is epidemic. Opioid overdoses have driven down life expectancy in the USA for two consecutive years. We are also seeking high-tech medical fixes for diseases of lifestyle: obesity, diabetes, cardiovascular disease, alcoholism and depression. We have lost sight of the origins of illness and wellness and are fixated on sophisticated and expensive medical patch-ups.

A

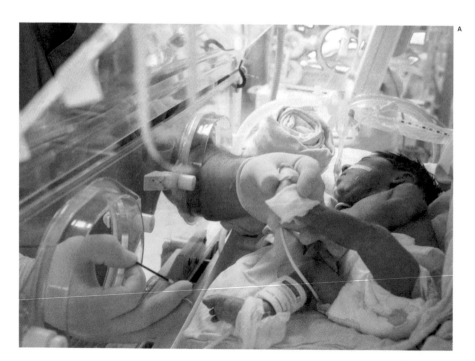

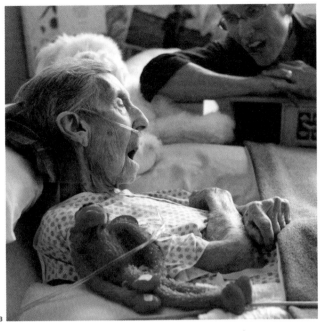

A Prenatal care is offered at the ISSS hospital in San Salvador. Medical interventions at the beginning of life have led to enormous reductions in infant and maternal mortality and can be counted among medicine's major success stories.

B A terminally ill patient receives care at the now-closed Hospice of Saint John in Lakewood, Colorado. It accepted patients regardless of their ability to pay, although most were covered by Medicare or Medicaid. Ensuring access to proper end of life care offers particular challenges for systems that rely on insurance and private payment.

B

Medicine is also spreading into more and more areas of life. Much of what was once thought, albeit ruefully, to be part of the human condition has become a medical, and therefore treatable, disorder. Childbirth, the psychological transitions of adolescence, shyness, unhappiness, baldness, even ageing – they are all increasingly medical phenomena. This can bring enormous benefits – 'natural' childbirth could be deadly – but also searching questions: what is ordinary human functioning and what is a medical condition? Given that few medical interventions are risk-free, what should we live with and when should we turn to medicine for relief? Death is ceasing to be the inevitable, if bitterly unwelcome, end of things, and is becoming a medical failure. All too often we die in intensive treatment units, rigged to unsleeping machines, medicated, catheterized, traumatized. Life is exquisitely valuable, but is this how we want it to close? Is this a blessing?

Increasingly, medicine also does more than treat the sick. We treat the well in anticipation of future disease. This certainly seems sensible: go upstream; prevention is better than cure. But is medical prevention always better?

The medical skirmish over prescribing statins for lowering LDL cholesterol in the asymptomatic has raised important questions: can the anticipated benefits of treatment justify the predictable side effects? By medicating the well, are we extending lives or massively increasing the population of the sick? And shouldn't we be prioritizing non-medical prevention: exercise, good nutrition, giving up smoking? Is Western medicine still good for us? Although its achievements are unparalleled, it is less certain that we have got the balance right. For decades the beneficiaries of medicine's extraordinary successes, we are in danger of becoming its victims.

Are we still certain we are doing more good than harm?

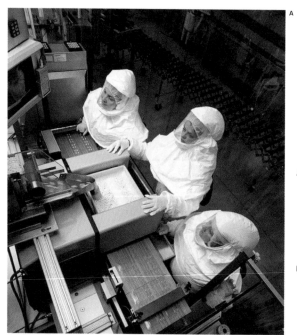

A

LDL cholesterol
Low-density lipoprotein cholesterol. Frequently referred to as 'bad cholesterol' and associated, at high levels, with heart disease.

A Workers monitor the production of drugs in a factory. Although modern pharmaceuticals can deliver benefits, the pharmaceutical industry is a powerful driver of 'medicalization', bringing more and more aspects of human life under a medical purview. And all drugs have side effects.
B A worker on the production line checks the labelling on a pharmaceutical bottle. Increasingly, medical and pharmaceutical interventions seek to improve on ordinary well-being, or to anticipate and ward off future ill health.

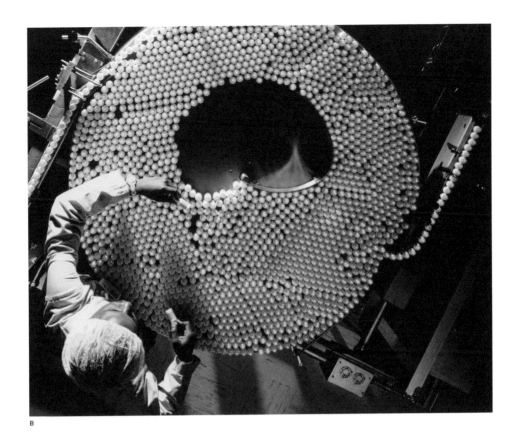

B

The purview of medicine is also expanding beyond ordinary good health. It no longer restricts itself to the prevention and treatment of disease.

Where once it launched assaults on brutal killers – cholera, tuberculosis, polio – it has become increasingly possible to improve on well-being. Why restrict ourselves to the prevention of disease when, with the same technologies, we can improve on ordinary functioning? If drugs for those with attention deficits can quicken the minds of those considered normal, why not take them? And given how highly we rate mental excellence, why not make these drugs obligatory? Shouldn't we give them to schoolchildren alongside their iPads and textbooks?

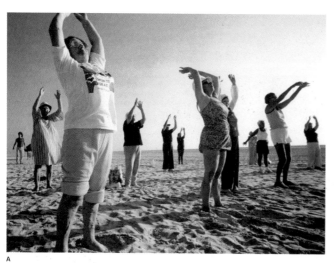

A   Elderly people take an early morning exercise class at Miami Beach, Florida, in 1985. Despite all the brilliance of high-tech medicine, exercise remains a cornerstone of good health.

B   Saudi Civil Defense members use a forklift to move Khaled Shaeri, aged 20, from his house in Jazan, to be airlifted to Riyadh for medical treatment. In 2013, Shaeri weighed approximately 1,345 pounds (610 kg) and was suffering from severe obesity due to health problems. Tackling 'obesogenic' environments and overcoming barriers to activity and healthy nutrition are urgent and increasingly global public health challenges.

A

Furthermore, medicine has not drawn a boundary at the living. Genetic engineering raises the possibility of trans-generational change, of both designing out unwanted features and designing in desirable ones. Although no sane person would mourn the passing of Huntington's chorea, once we move away from the grossest disorders, we encounter deep and fraught questions: given the enormous benefits of human diversity, can we say, with confidence, what is and is not desirable? And who should make such momentous decisions? Medical technology can lead us a long way from the compassionate treatment of the sick.

Among the most urgent questions is how are we to afford it all?

Every country in the world struggles to meet the escalating costs of health care. The causes of these rising costs are complex. Partly, they stem from medicine's phenomenal success. With the routing of the old killer infectious diseases, better nutrition, improved sanitation and healthier environments, life expectancy, in the West at least, has leapt. But longevity opens the door to the diseases of ageing. Seldom curable in the ordinary sense, they can require years of increasingly expensive medical support. With age, co-morbidities can proliferate, and polypharmacy is often the expensive and not always desirable result.

Affluence has brought its own morbidities. 'Want' – first in the list of evils (disease, ignorance, squalor and idleness followed) drawn up by Sir William Beveridge (1879–1963) in 1942 – has retreated, in the West at least. People are seldom famished. But 'plenty' has brought soaring levels of obesity with their attendant disorders: diabetes, musculo-skeletal problems, cardiovascular disease. These appear to be, in part, the result of our powerful economies. The food industry delivers mass-produced and highly processed foods at low cost. There is also our increasingly 'obesogenic' environment. Not only are we surrounded by cheap and calorific food, but we also drive or take public transport where once we would have walked. Working life is increasingly sedentary; leisure time is often spent in front of screens. Our comforts are killing us.

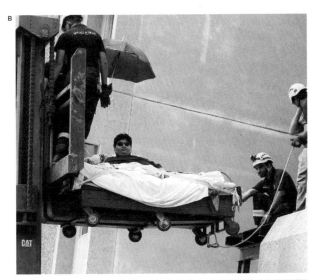

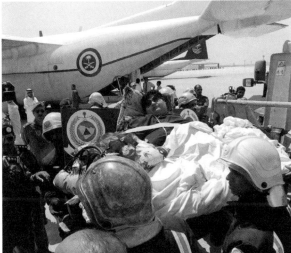

Huntington's chorea
Also known as Huntington's disease. A genetically inherited degenerative disorder of the brain and nervous system that leads to dementia and death.

Polypharmacy Usually taken to mean the simultaneous prescription of multiple drugs to individuals. Although at times medically indicated, the term 'polypharmacy' is often used pejoratively to describe over-treatment, particularly among older patients.

'Obesogenic' environment
Refers loosely to the tendency of many modern environments to encourage the consumption of unhealthy and excessively calorific food and to make it difficult for people to take exercise.

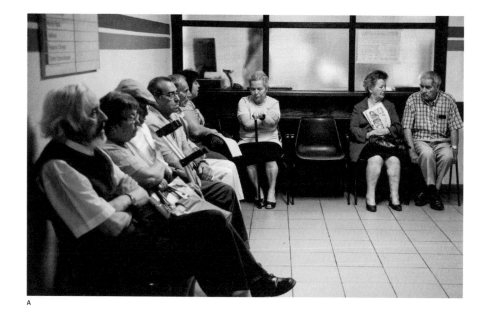

A

There are also steeply rising patient expectations. We want to feel better, live longer, be happier – and so we turn to medicine. When we see a doctor, we expect treatment: for stressed doctors and expectant patients, the prescription pad is often where the consultation ends, despite the self-limiting nature of many ordinary ailments.

Then there is the medical-industrial complex. Clinical practice is sustained by a network of powerful corporations seeking markets for their goods and services. Some of this brings benefits. But corporations go in search of profits. The wider the scope of medicine, the more conditions that become treatable, the louder patients clamour for treatment, the better the profits. As a result, the costs of medicine rise inexorably, outstripping our ability to pay.

A Patients sit in the São José Hospital waiting room in Lisbon during a two-day doctors' strike in July 2012. The tensions in modern health care between costs, expectations and the interests of health professionals make medicine a global political flashpoint.

B Landing page for Ping An Good Doctor, a commercial Chinese online health platform. Health care is a huge global business, but when patients pay for services it raises important questions about justice: those without resources cannot get access to good health care.

In addition, there is a crisis of confidence in medicine. Trust, so central to the doctor-patient relationship, is being eroded. Partly, this is to do with increasing awareness of medicine's fallibility; partly, the rise of the information age and expert patients. But patients can feel lost in the hyper-specialized fields of modern medicine, their experience of illness dissolved into the arcane language of biochemical science.

There is nothing inevitable about the direction Western medicine has taken. What is good and necessary is not welded to its downside. Medicine, once unambiguously good for us, can be good for us again. But it must change.

Medical-industrial complex
General term for the network of commercial companies that provide health goods and services. Concerns are often raised about the impact of profit-seeking behaviour by large corporations on the sustainability of health services.

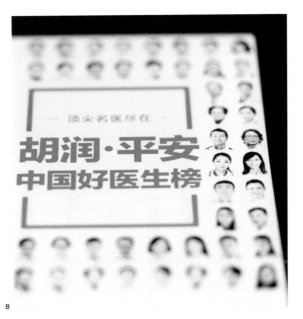

B

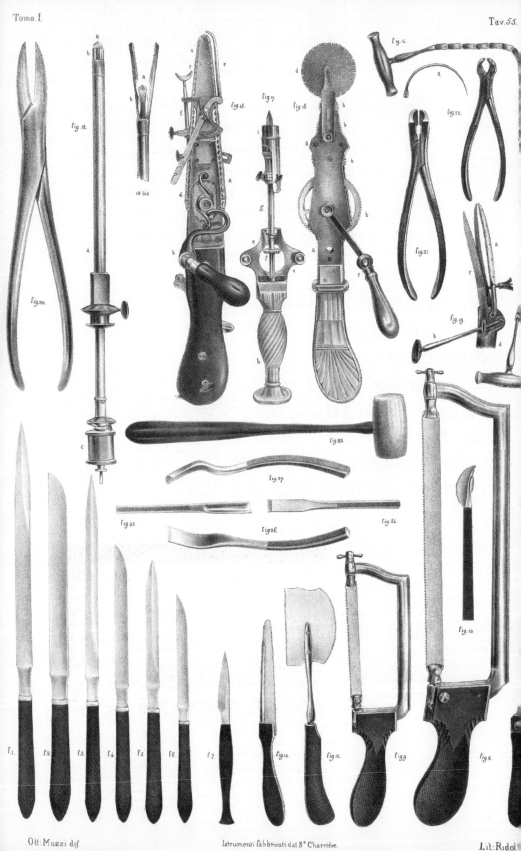

Istrumenti fabbricati dal S.ʳ Charrière.

1. The Development of Medicine

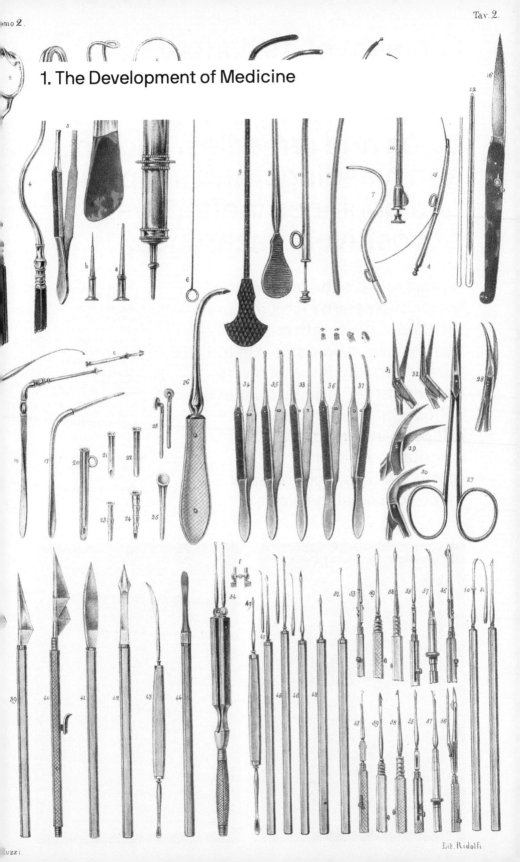

For most of its history, Western medicine has been almost entirely useless – its cures and remedies, cuppings and bleedings, and simples and poultices ineffective or positively hazardous.

Hippocrates is the undisputed father of Western medicine, and the Hippocratic oath may be the best-known medical text in the West. Allegedly, it is still sworn on graduation at some medical schools, although presumably adapted: in some translations, it contains an injunction to refrain from seducing slaves in the houses of the sick.

A This 11th-century English miniature depicts an operation to remove haemorrhoids (right). A patient with gout is treated with cutting and burning of the feet (left).

B Although often dramatic, many early medical interventions were almost entirely useless, such as this cupping therapy seen in *Ophthalmodouleia* by Georg Bartisch (1583).

C A medical staple for centuries, bloodletting was eventually shown to be ineffective. From *Li Livres dou Santé* by Aldobrandino of Siena (late 13th century).

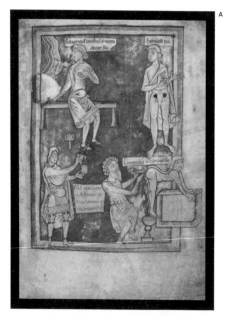

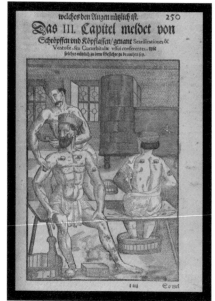

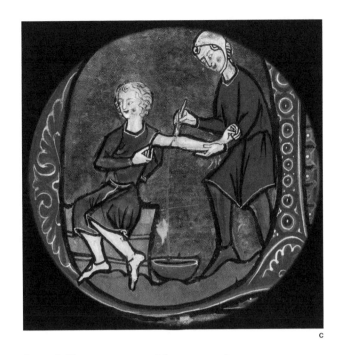

c

Medicine, from its Hippocratic roots until the mid-19th century, was little more than a way to distract the patient while waiting to see if they recovered. According to French philosopher Voltaire (1694–1778), doctors 'were men who put drugs of which they know little, to cure diseases of which they know less, into bodies of which they know nothing at all'. Some of this changed, and dramatically, from the mid-19th century onwards. But not all of it. As the great medical historian Roy Porter (1946–2002) wrote: 'The prominence of medicine has lain only in small measure in its ability to make the sick well. This was always true, and remains so today.'

Hippocratic medicine was naturalistic. Unlike many of the belief systems of the ancient Near East, it did not look for the origins of disease in divine displeasure, supernatural intervention or dark magic. Health and illness were *natural* phenomena, amenable to observation and reason. Man was subject to the same natural laws as the rest of the universe and could be understood accordingly.

A   In the *Corpus Hippocraticum*, health was a balance of the four humours or *chymoi*, and poor health came from their imbalance. Here, Byrhtferth's diagram, from a 12th-century manuscript, indicates that the humours were regarded as part of the natural order of the universe.

B   In the Middle Ages, barbers did more than cut hair; they were also surgeons. As the *Guild Book of the Barber Surgeons of York* (1486) shows, medieval surgery combined anatomy, astrology and religion. Surgeons calculated the moon's position before surgery.

Hippocratic medicine was also holistic and patient-centred. The Hippocratic doctor needed a thorough understanding of how his patients lived and worked, what they ate and drank, what we call their 'family history'. Healing involved careful watching and investigation of the individual patient: empiricism was stronger than theory.

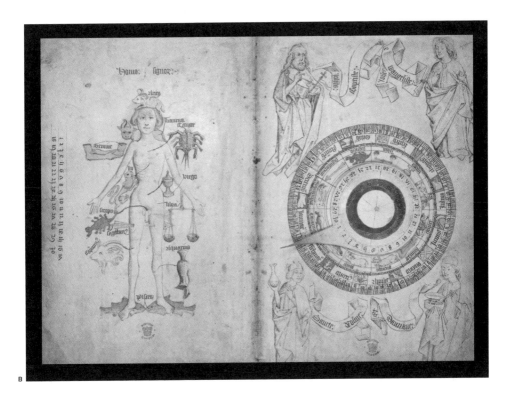

B

At the centre of the *Corpus Hippocraticum* lies the concept of the humours or *chymoi* (translated as juice or sap). The humours can be thought of as the constitutive fluids of the human body – the origin of all our other fluids. *On the Nature of Man* (440–400 BCE, part of the *Corpus Hippocraticum* although usually attributed to Polybus), states: 'The human body contains blood, phlegm, yellow bile and black bile. These are the things that make up its constitution and cause its pains and health. Health is primarily that state in which these constituent substances are in the correct proportion to each other, both in strength and quantity, and are well mixed. Pain occurs when one of the substances presents either a deficiency or an excess, or is separated in the body and not mixed with others.'

Humours According to humoral theory, the human body consists of four humours – blood, yellow bile, black bile and phlegm. Each has its corresponding element – air, fire, earth and water – and its associated property – hot, dry, cold and wet. Each has an associated organ: blood with the heart; yellow bile with the liver; black bile with the spleen and phlegm with the brain. Each also has an associated temperament: blood makes a person sanguine or optimistic; yellow bile turns one choleric or irascible. Black bile is associated with melancholy and phlegm with imperturbability or calm.

Holistic Medicine that aims to treat the whole person, looking at aspects of emotional, psychological and spiritual well-being. Sometimes it is opposed to 'allopathic' medicine, which targets the individual disease.

Empiricism The theory that all knowledge of the world is derived from the senses. Associated with the rise of experimental science, it privileges direct experience of the world over theory or established authority.

It is likely that observing the fluids discharged during illness contributed to humoral medicine. Colds and diarrhoea saw an excessive flow from the body; fevers saw sweating and flushing. Certain illnesses brought changes to urine and faeces. Blood turned dark, almost black, when it dried. Humoral medicine offered a simple but compelling schema that was not seriously challenged until the 18th century and not replaced until the 19th.

Despite the distance in time, the paucity of Greek anatomical knowledge and the varied nature of the writings attributed to him, Hippocrates still speaks to modern disputes. His focus on the whole person, not the isolated disease or dysfunction, has seen him championed by supporters of 'family medicine' and by complementary and alternative therapists.

In Hippocrates, we also find the essential medical triad: the relationship between the doctor, the patient and the disease.

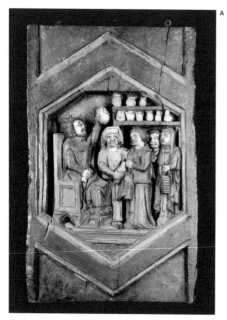
A

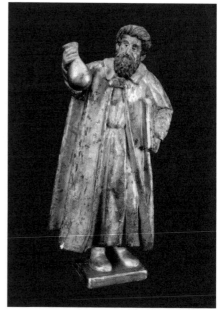
B

A   In this painted relief after Giotto, a medical practitioner examines urine brought by his patients. The effect of illnesses on bodily excretions, such as urine and faeces, may have contributed to the development of humoral theory.

B   This wooden statue (1770–1850) shows St Cosmas, patron saint of druggists, surgeons and dentists, performing uroscopy: studying a patient's urine was said to provide information about the state of their humours.

C   Urine wheels were used for diagnosing diseases based on the colour, smell and taste of a patient's urine. This example, from *Epiphanie Medicorum* (1506) by Ullrich Pinder, was used for diagnosing metabolic diseases.

c

This triad remains central to medicine, but the emphasis given to each element shifts with different medical eras. Today, some find that the intense focus on disease, manifest in super-specialization (the division of body and mind into an ever-increasing proliferation of sub-specialties) dehumanizes medicine and alienates us from our own health and well-being. The concept of 'balance', although semantically elastic, still has its place in modern medicine: we talk of a balanced diet, of a biological system's equilibrium or homeostasis.

The second medical colossus of the ancient world is Galen of Pergamum.

A Greek of the Roman Empire, Galen was a prolific and combative medical writer and philosopher. A brilliant self-publicist, and court physician to the Stoic emperor Marcus Aurelius (121–180 CE), Galen was the supreme medical authority in Western medicine for more than a millennium. He systematized the Hippocratic legacy – most practitioners met Hippocrates through Galen – and added to it knowledge of anatomy and physiology, acquired through animal dissection.

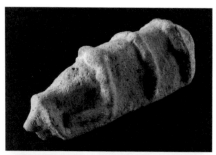

A

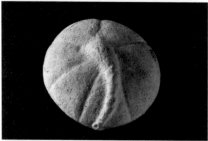

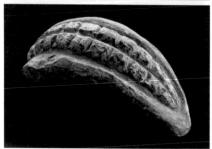

Galen of Pergamum (129–c. 216 CE) After Hippocrates, Galen is the second most important physician of the ancient world. His huge body of work systematized and popularized the Hippocratic legacy.

A Empirical and religious approaches to illnesses were frequently blended in pre-Modern Europe. Roman votive offerings (top to bottom: trachea, placenta, teeth and mouth) were left at healing sanctuaries by those seeking healing from divine intervention. Usually depicting the site of illness, these naturalistic offerings were a form of sympathetic magic.
B This display shows replicas of Roman surgical instruments. They indicate that, alongside requests for divine intervention, Roman medicine was often intensely practical.

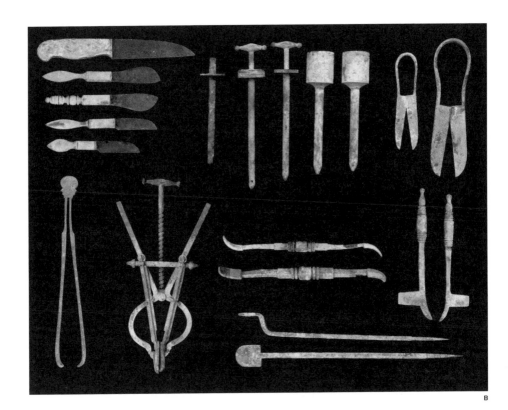

B

Although the use of anatomical investigations to understand how bodies worked would have profound implications for medicine, human dissection was taboo in the ancient world: the cutting open of human corpses was largely banned in both ancient Greece and Rome and was subsequently forbidden by the Church. Forced to draw largely on animal models, Galen made mistakes, and given his stature these had repercussions for more than 1,000 years. It was not until the 14th century, when human dissections became more common, that knowledge of the inner workings of the human body began to gather pace.

Most medieval Europeans took their healing where they found it: from faith healers, herb gatherers, adepts and family elders. But academic medicine was largely preoccupied with fitting the theoretical models of the great authorities – Hippocrates and Galen – to the messy reality of human disease. Loyalty to Galenic theory took priority over learning from clinical experience. As a result, empiricism, the belief that evidence and experience provide true knowledge of the world, waned.

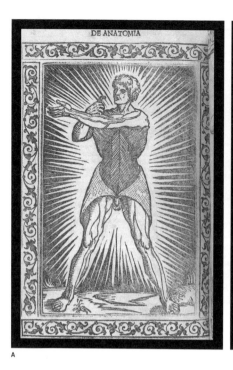
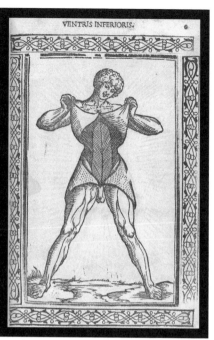

A

Then came the Renaissance. Scholars disagree over its origins and timing, but from the 14th century the intellectual life of Europe was transformed. In one sense, the Renaissance involved a return to the authority and prestige of ancient Greece and Rome, partly invigorated by re-translations of Arabic versions of classical texts. This was a return to the sparkling, semi-miraculous sources of Western civilization. And yet the Renaissance was also marked by irresistible curiosity about the world as it is. Empiricism was as much a pillar of the Renaissance as a reverence for classical authority. (Among the origins of the word 'empiricism' is the Greek *empeirikos* – a doctor who relies on evidence alone.)

A Prohibitions on autopsy were swept away and direct anatomical observation of the human body challenged aspects of Galenic authority and led to a huge increase in empirical knowledge. Anatomical illustration from a work by Jacopo Berengario da Carpi (1523).

B The publication by Andreas Vesalius of *On the Fabric of the Human Body* (1543) established anatomy as the superior empirical medical science and helped overthrow Galenic orthodoxy.

It was only a matter of time before the new investigations started questioning classical authority. Nowhere was this more obvious than in the opening, figuratively and literally, of the human body. Medieval prohibitions against human dissection were brushed aside.

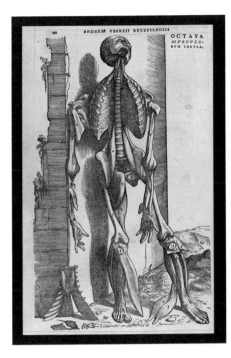

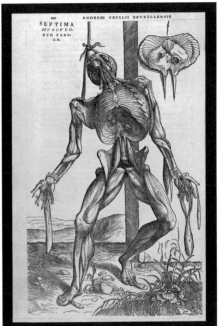

B

Before the 14th century, autopsy was unusual.

Most dissections were performed on animals and were regarded as secondary illustrations of indisputable Galenic authority. In *c.* 1315, the first recorded public dissection was performed in Bologna by the Italian physician, anatomist and professor of surgery Mondino de' Luzzi, also known as Mundinus (*c.* 1270–1326).

Autopsy Literally 'go and look for yourself'. From the Greek *autos* (self) and *opsis* (sight). Now refers to a thorough surgical investigation of a body by dissection to identify the cause of death or the presence of pathology.

The true founder of modern anatomy though is the Belgian physician Andreas Vesalius (1514–64), author of *On the Fabric of the Human Body* (1543). The publication established anatomy as the descriptive medical science par excellence and the jewel in the medical crown for centuries. Although Vesalius was hugely influenced by Galen, he began to transcend the master and pointed out errors arising from Galen's reliance on animal corpses: the lower human jaw was a single bone, not two; the human liver does not have five lobes. Empiricism was on the march.

If the Renaissance was the great bridge between medieval and modern Europe, another critical stage, gathering pace in the late Renaissance and reaching into the Enlightenment, is the scientific revolution, without which modernity is inconceivable.

Its most spectacular achievements were in astronomy and cosmology, and Sir Isaac Newton (1642–1727) its apotheosis. It arrived with the publication, by Nicolaus Copernicus (1473–1543), of *On the Revolutions of the Heavenly Spheres* (1543).

Inevitably, the scientific revolution was felt in medicine, largely through developments in chemistry and physics. Among the pioneers was the Swiss physician Paracelsus (1493–1541). More mystic than scientist, his influence was two-fold: he wanted to cast off the burden of ancient authority and found medicine on modern principles, and he looked to chemistry to explain how the body works, to identify maladies and to find cures. His work on the digestive origins of uric crystals and kidney stones was an early attempt to identify the chemical origins of illness. Paracelsus, for all his contradictions and love of mysticism and esoterica, believed passionately that the road to truth lay through experiment and observation. Go and look for yourself.

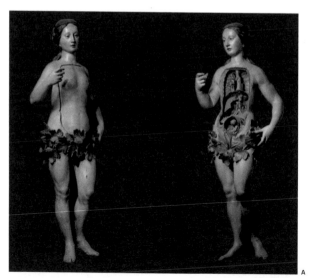

A   As human bodies for dissection were in short supply, models such as this 17th-century anatomical Eve were developed to help teach students – and interested others – the basic principles of human anatomy. These anatomical models reached extraordinary heights of sophistication in the 18th century, although many modern viewers find the juxtaposition of female beauty with revealed viscera unsettling.

B   It was not until the 17th century that Sir William Harvey established categorically that the heart is a pump that drives the blood in ceaseless circulation around the human body. This drawing of the mitral valve is from Richard Lower's *Tractatus de Corde* (1669).

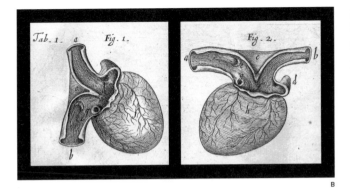
B

Scientific revolution
Refers loosely to a time of intellectual transformation during the European Early Modern period that saw the emergence of techniques of investigation and understanding that characterize modern science. Although its timing is debated, it is often said to have been inaugurated by the publication of Copernicus' *On the Revolutions of the Heavenly Spheres* in 1543.

Ontologically separate
Refers to a discrete and separate entity existing independently of the body. Usually thought of as entering the body and bringing about a diseased state or condition. A clear example is the 'germ' theory of disease. Ontological theory can be contrasted to humoral theory, which sees illness as the expression of an imbalance in the humours.

Medicine had its own Copernican revolution, courtesy of the English physician Sir William Harvey (1578–1657) and his discovery of the heart-driven circulation of the blood. Using dissection and direct observation, Harvey overthrew the Galenic consensus. In his landmark *On the Motion of the Heart and Blood* (1628), he stated: 'It is absolutely necessary to conclude that the blood in the animal body is impelled in a circle and is in a state of ceaseless motion.' The human body, like the heavens, was yielding secrets unfathomed by the ancients to modern investigation.

Together with investigation went classification. Where the Hippocratic tradition had tended to see illnesses as specific – to individuals, temperaments and environments – the new science increasingly saw diseases as ontologically separate: discrete entities distinct from their sufferers. This shift would have enormous consequences.

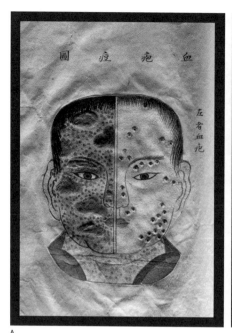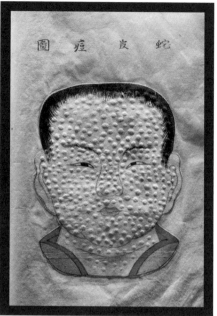

A

The tension between a focus on the disease entity and the patient's experience of illness remains a flashpoint in medicine.

The Enlightenment passion for classification achieved its apotheosis in the work of the Swedish naturalist Carl von Linné, better known as Linnaeus (1707–78). His binomial system of classification named the natural world, and its success led to attempts to bring the same classificatory rigour to medicine. The 18th century saw the development of a range of nosologies – systems of disease classification – including those by Scottish physician William Cullen (1710–90) and English physician Erasmus Darwin (1731–1802).

Despite the optimism and intellectual curiosity of Enlightenment thought, medicine remained therapeutically stunted.

A The 18th century saw an intense interest in the classification of diseases. This representation of smallpox is from a Japanese manuscript (1720) by Kanda Gensen.

B Tuberculosis was a terrible killer, particularly associated with the insanitary conditions of 19th-century urban slums. Illustration of pulmonary TB (1834) by Samuel G. Moreton.

There were exceptions – inoculation against smallpox, quinine for malaria – but the therapeutic cupboard was shockingly bare. Anatomy had revealed the secrets of the body's functioning and diseases were becoming better understood, but cures remained infuriatingly elusive. It was not until the 19th century and the rise of hospital-based medicine that the battle against illness started to shift, gradually at first but with increasing rapidity, in humankind's favour.

After the French Revolution of 1789, the centre of Western medicine moved decisively to France. The revolutionary government inaugurated a new systematic, scientific, hands-on approach, and at its heart were the great Paris hospitals. They were vast. There were more beds (20,000) in Paris hospitals at the beginning of the 19th century than in England. Mostly, patients were drawn from the uneducated and powerless urban poor. Doctors had access to enormous numbers of clinical cases, to what easily came, in these impersonal institutions, to be called clinical *material.* Many of them were suffering from diseases associated with urban poverty and overcrowding. Infectious diseases, particularly tuberculosis and typhoid, were endemic.

Endemic A disease is said to be endemic when it is established in a steady state for a given population in a specific area. It can be contrasted with epidemic, which refers to the rapid spread of a disease to a large number of people in a given population, usually over a relatively short period of time.

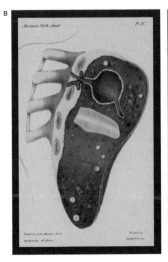

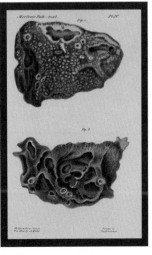

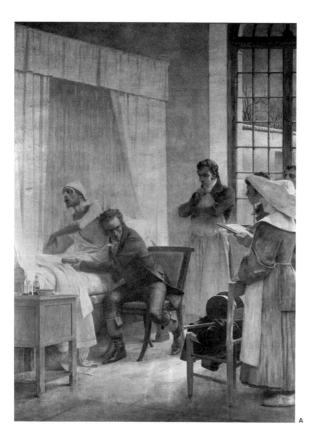

A

Before the rise of modern hospital medicine, the paradigm of the clinical encounter was between a physician and his – it was almost always 'his' – patient. Illness and disease were seen as highly personal, an expression of the relationship between the patient and the environment.

The physician's role was to interrogate the riddle.

Paris medicine synthesized a new, enormously influential approach. At its heart was the lesion, the unmistakeable biomarker of pathological change. Visible by its effects, or directly under a microscope, disease developed a new objective existence. Doctors were encouraged to look for these objective signs rather than relying on patient accounts. Increasingly, following diagnosis in the living, the presence of pathology was corroborated after death, via autopsy. The morgue was as essential as the hospital to French medicine.

To the identification of pathological change was added the importance of statistics. The French hospitals dealt with vast numbers of the sick. With so many people ill, and so little knowledge of what worked, hospital medicine, allied to Enlightenment quantification, made possible the numerical assessment of outcomes. Paris saw the forerunner of the modern clinical trial. Using these techniques, Pierre Louis (1787–1872) overturned therapeutic bloodletting, which had been a medical staple for millennia. He showed that it made absolutely no difference to the progress of pneumonia whether blood was taken early or late, in large or small amounts.

Although therapeutic advances were slow in the first half of the 19th century, Paris laid the ground for modern diagnostic techniques. There were three essentials.

First, physical diagnosis following clinical inspection. Along with careful looking, this would usually involve one or more of the three diagnostic arts: palpation (touch), percussion (tapping) and auscultation (listening). Second, the use of post-mortem examination to identify pathological change. Third, numerical analysis. The huge numbers of sick people permitted the accumulation of massive amounts of data about specific diseases.

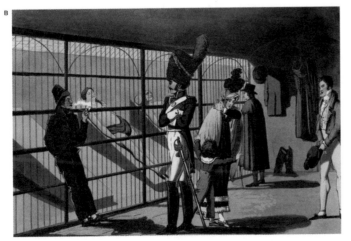

B

Pathology The study of disease. From the Greek *pathos* (disease) and *logos* (discourse). A pathologist is a doctor who specializes in the study of diseases. Pathology is also used to refer to the disease itself.

For all its clinical brilliance, its systematization and its identification of the pathological roots of illness, Paris medicine came with a cost.

Medicine became increasingly focused on individual pathology at the expense of the patient. Diseases were abstracted from the people who suffered them and the environments that helped precipitate them. The power imbalance between doctors and their frequently uneducated patients hardened. Medicine became welded to that most paradoxical of modern institutions, the hospital.

A   The conditions of the urban poor living in industrial cities such as Glasgow (here photographed by Thomas Annan in 1868) led to appalling health outcomes. Poor sanitation and nutrition were significant killers.

B   In the 1890s, Jacob A. Riis documented the urban slums of New York, where rates of child mortality were catastrophic. Overcrowding meant that infectious diseases spread rapidly. On the right, lodgers are renting 'spots' for five cents.

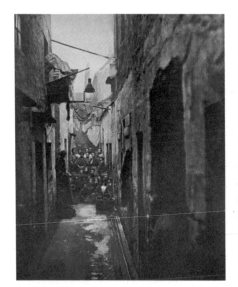

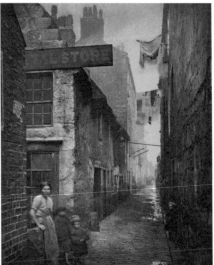

A

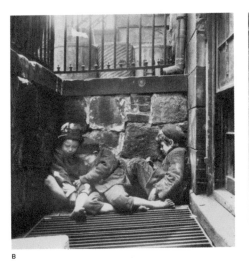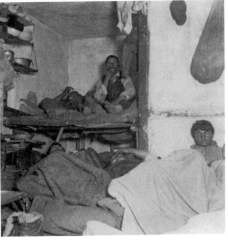

B

Despite the decisive shift of clinical scientific medicine to the hospital, the most dramatic improvements were associated with changes in public health: the health of populations, rather than individuals.

The growth – in Europe, the USA and Japan – of 19th-century industrial cities, the arrival of large numbers of rural poor (in 1750 about 15% of the population of Britain lived in towns; by 1880 it was 80%) and their concentration in urban slums in conditions of appalling squalor led to catastrophic health outcomes. Rates of child and infant mortality soared; life expectancy dipped below the 20s in some areas. Malnutrition, lack of sanitation, overcrowding, industrial accidents and disease took an appalling toll. Rickets, typhoid, typhus, tuberculosis, diphtheria, scarlet fever, measles, chicken pox and of course cholera all bred in the filth of the industrial slums. In 1832, some 7,000 people died in London during a cholera outbreak. In Russia, between 1847 and 1861, cholera killed more than a million people.

Philanthropy aside, there were strong incentives for the powerful to take an interest. Diseases that bred in the slums did not stay in the slums: they threatened genteel lives. There were strong links between pauperism, unemployment and ill health: sickness imposed a costly burden on the state.

In 1842, the English social reformer Edwin Chadwick (1800–90) published his *Report on the Sanitary Condition of the Labouring Population of Great Britain*. Chadwick laid the blame for illnesses of poverty on insanitary living conditions. He subscribed to the prevalent miasmatic theory of disease, whose origins lay in the fetid emanations of decomposition and filth. His solution: drainage, refuse collection and clean water.

In 1854, while investigating an outbreak of cholera in Soho, the surgeon John Snow (1813–58) identified its source in the Broad Street water pump. Although the outbreak was in decline, when the parish guardians removed the pump handle, the number of cases fell. Snow's theory was confirmed: cholera was waterborne. Like Chadwick, Snow pressed for major changes to sanitation and water supply. The summer of 1858 also brought London's 'great stink'. So foul was the stench from the Thames – little more than an open sewer – that despite Parliament soaking its curtains in chloride of lime, proceedings had to be suspended. The result was the hasty funding of Joseph Bazalgette's (1819–91) sewers and the construction of the Thames embankment to improve the river's flow.

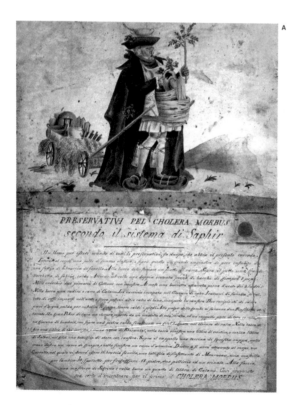

A

Miasmatic theory of disease Now obsolete, miasmatic theory held that the origin of diseases lay in 'bad' or polluted air – also referred to as 'night air' – given off by decaying organic matter. Effectively replaced by germ theory.

A   Water supplies were frequently contaminated by human faeces and were a source of lethal cholera epidemics. Here, a man from Nuremberg sports a variety of quack remedies and protections to ward off the 1832 cholera epidemic, which killed up to 7,000 people in London alone.
B   The scourge of cholera and other infectious diseases led to the development of increased public health surveillance and control by the state. Developments in microbiology were a critical part of this process. In 1849, the General Board of Health published this cholera map of London.
C   London's 'great stink' of 1858 led to the temporary closure of Parliament and the funding of a vast new sewage system. Here, the Northern Outfall sewer – the largest in London – is under construction, supervised by Joseph Bazalgette (top right).

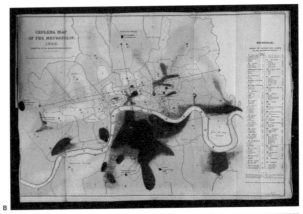

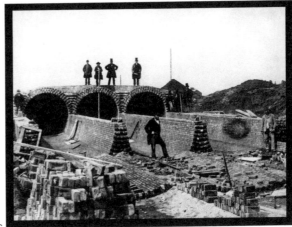

Although earlier public health measures, piecemeal and of uncertain effectiveness, had been developed – usually to contain apocalyptic visitations of the plague, such as the *cordon sanitaire* imposed between Austria and the Ottoman Empire in 1770 – something like a modern public health infrastructure, complete, in some cases, with considerable coercive power, was developed in many Western countries from the middle decades of the 19th century.

Increasingly, health was no longer just a personal matter – it was subject to the scrutiny, and where necessary the force, of the state.

Microbiology The study of organisms too small to be seen by the human eye. As an emerging discipline, it made important contributions to the identification of the origins of many diseases in pathogenic micro-organisms.

Attenuated vaccine A vaccine created by attenuating, or reducing the virulence, of a pathogen. It provokes an immune response in the human body without initiating a full-blown episode of the disease, thereby conferring ongoing immunity.

Towards the end of the century, the new state structures of public health were drawing some of their justification, and much of their effectiveness, from the impact of developments in microbiology. Medicine was beginning to flex its therapeutic muscles.

The idea that unseen micro-organisms lay behind disease was not novel; talk of 'animalcules' (microscopic animals) and 'fomites' (infectious material) long preceded laboratory identification. Furthermore, inoculation against smallpox – provoking a mild form of the disease in healthy individuals to bring about immunity – went back to 10th-century China. However, it was not until Louis Pasteur (1822–95) in France and Robert Koch (1843–1910) in Germany that the microbial origins of many common diseases started to be identified.

A

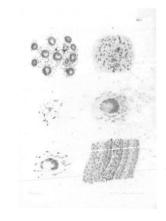
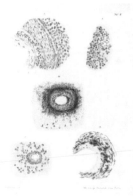
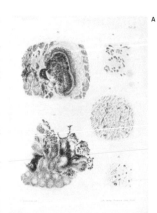

A scientist rather than a doctor, Pasteur initially tackled agricultural problems. He identified the organism responsible for souring wine and showed that heating it to between 50 and 60 degrees Celsius – pasteurization – overcame the problem. He then developed a vaccine for avian cholera: infecting healthy chickens with 'stale' microbes provoked immunity. Using the anthrax bacillus identified by Koch, he developed an 'attenuated' vaccine against a disease that decimated French livestock. More remarkable still was his rabies vaccination. A virus rather than a microbe, the infectious agent was invisible to the microscope, so he did not know the agent he was dealing with. Recognizing that the symptoms of the disease suggested it attacked the nervous system, he used the spinal cords of rabbits to develop an attenuated vaccine effective against animals, and in July 1885, to enormous acclaim, he successfully treated a nine-year-old boy.

Meanwhile, Pasteur's great rival Koch identified the causative agents of tuberculosis – a disease long attributed to environment and constitution – and the dreaded cholera. His methodical research practices established bacteriology as a discipline and confirmed the germ theory of disease. In the years between 1879 and 1900, bacteriologists identified the agents responsible for most serious infectious diseases.

A   Tuberculosis – also known as consumption – was among the most feared and symbolically charged diseases of the 19th century. However, revolutionary improvements in the science of microbiology started to transform understanding of the major infectious diseases. In 1882, the great German microbiologist Robert Koch published his findings on tuberculosis in *Die Aetiologie der Tuberkulose* (*The Etiology of Tuberculosis*). He identified the causative agent of tuberculosis: the slow-growing *Mycobacterium tuberculosis*. These illustrations are from the 1884 edition of his work.

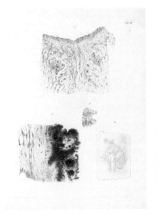
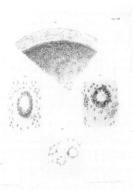
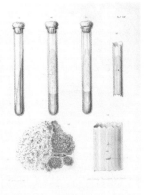

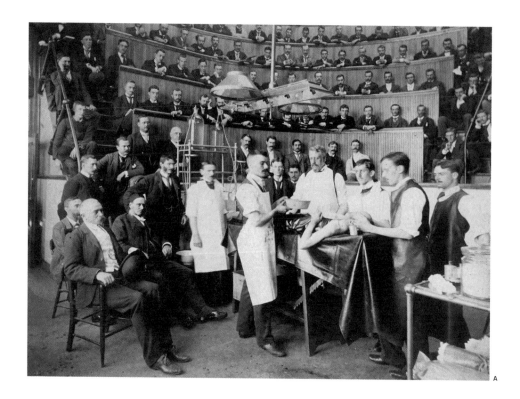

A

Germ theory transformed surgical practice.

Surgical history is not for the faint hearted. Before the introduction of anaesthetic in the 1840s, surgery was brutal, painful and usually fatal. If the trauma didn't kill the patient, infection usually obliged. Although the new anaesthesia helped the pain, mortality from post-operative infection was still appalling.

Drawing on Pasteur's research, the English surgeon Joseph Lister (1827–1912) started using carbolic as a disinfecting agent, with improved outcomes. With the germ origins of infection identified, the use of antiseptic agents rapidly gave way to asepsis: the exclusion of as much bacteria as possible using sterile equipment and hygienic methods. Although surgery was transformed, sloughing off its lowly status and, by the end of the 19th century, acquiring some of its contemporary glamour, it remained controversial. Mortality and post-operative complications were significant. Surgery was largely unregulated, and some surgeons were cavalier, removing lengths of bowel as a 'cure' for constipation. In the early 20th century, tonsillectomies were effectively a 'cure all' for recurrent childhood infections. Despite its risks, surgery became the default intervention.

The final contribution of germ theory came with the isolation of penicillin by bacteriologist Alexander Fleming (1881–1955). It was an accidental discovery. Fleming had been studying staphylococci, the microbes responsible for infections such as sepsis and pneumonia. In 1928, returning from holiday, he noticed that a mould had formed on a Petri dish in his lab and destroyed the staphylococci. It was penicillin.

It was not until a decade or more later though, with the work of the Australian Howard Florey (1898–1968) and his team at Oxford, that the therapeutic benefits of penicillin began to be realized. In 1941, Florey extracted enough penicillin to try it on a patient: a policeman who had contracted septicaemia while pruning roses. Within days he was recovering – although, tragically, the penicillin ran out and he died. Production then moved to the USA, with extraordinary results: bacterial infection rates were slashed. Serious and often fatal infections such as pneumococcal pneumonia, bacterial meningitis and endocarditis could be treated.

Pneumonia was no longer a death sentence.

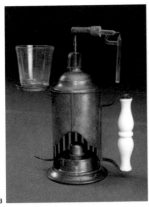
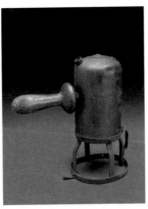

A   Modern medicine is inconceivable without the achievements of surgery, demonstrated here in the Paris School of Medicine operating theatre, 1890. However, therapeutic developments came late and depended on improvements in other areas, such as anaesthesia.

B   It was not until the introduction of disinfectants that mortality rates from surgery began to improve. Seen here is an early antiseptic spray with a glass nozzle.

C   Steam antiseptic sprays, such as this one by Joseph Lister, were designed to douse everyone and everything in the operating room with antiseptic carbolic acid.

The full therapeutic power of vaccination was also unleashed. Drawing on the work of Koch and Pasteur, scientists attacked some of the world's most vicious killers, with remarkable results. The list of diseases for which vaccinations were developed reads like a who's who of the apocalypse: polio, influenza, meningitis, diphtheria, hepatitis, measles. It is almost impossible to exaggerate the impact of these therapeutic advances, and we cannot calculate the number of lives saved. Medicine does the most miraculous things.

To therapeutics was added diagnostics.

X-rays, first identified in 1895 by the German physicist William Röntgen (1845–1923), were rapidly adapted for diagnostic purposes with steadily increasing sophistication. By the 1920s, chest X-rays had become routine. By the end of the 1960s, X-rays, combined with computing power, were providing three-dimensional images of internal anatomy, via the new computerized axial tomography (CAT) scans.

For the first time, therapeutic inroads were also made in mental illness.

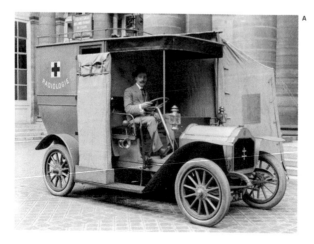

A

A   X-rays were rapidly adapted for diagnostic purposes, enabling doctors to get unparalleled views of the denser internal body structures such as bones. Seen here is a 1913 French mobile X-ray unit.

B   The 20th century saw the first inroads into the treatment of mental disorders, an area of human experience hitherto largely opaque to medicine. Some early interventions, such as electro-convulsive therapy, were, and remain, controversial. Here, a man is being treated for neuro-convulsive tremors with electro-therapy.

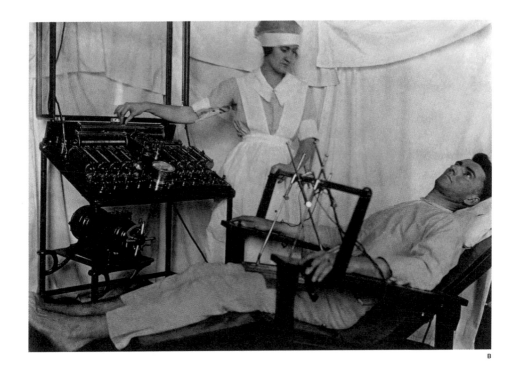

B

1949 saw the arrival of lithium: a powerful and effective psychotropic (mood or mind-altering) drug for the treatment of depression and bipolar disorder. More controversially, in the 1950s the first generation of antipsychotic drugs such as chlorpromazine came onto the market. Although effective at controlling some of the symptoms of major mental disorders, they had burdensome and stigmatizing neuro-muscular side effects such as Parkinsonism: trembling, sluggish movement, rigidity and loss of facial expression.

Computerized axial tomography (CAT) The development of three-dimensional pictures of internal body structures using X-rays from multiple angles that are then combined by powerful computers. Can show soft tissue structures invisible to ordinary X-rays.

In 1955, a chemist at Hoffmann-La Roche happened upon the first of what would become the most highly prescribed family of drugs in the 1960s, the anxiolytic (anxiety-reducing) benzodiazepines. The drug was first marketed in 1960 by Hoffmann-La Roche as Librium, followed in 1963 by Valium, one of the most highly prescribed drugs of all time. In the case of benzodiazepines though, early therapeutic optimism was replaced by serious concerns about dependency and side effects.

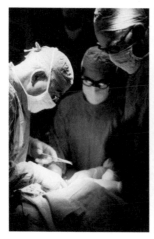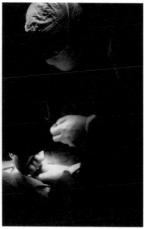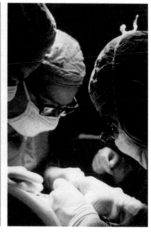

A

Post-war surgery was also transformed. In 1954, the first successful organ transplant – a kidney – took place in Boston, USA. As it was between identical twins, immune suppression was not necessary. Then, in 1967, the South African surgeon Christiaan Barnard (1922–2001) carried out the first heart transplant. Although the patient, Louis Washkansky, only lived for 18 days, Philip Blaiberg, Barnard's second patient, lived for nearly two years.

On the face of it, there appears to be no limit to medicine's technological powers. Still energized by the Enlightenment optimism of its golden age and having unravelled the secrets of DNA – supported by robust diagnostic tools and the analytical power of double-blind randomized controlled trials and big data – its therapeutic reach seems boundless. Even the immense mysteries of the human mind are yielding to neuroscience and its neuro-imaging techniques.

There is talk of spectacular longevity, even immortality.

But old problems remain and new ones are emerging with frightening speed. Infectious diseases have been replaced as major killers by diseases of lifestyle: obesity, diabetes, some cancers, heart disease.

A   After anaesthesia and asepsis, antibiotics further improved surgical outcomes. Increased knowledge of the immune system and the development of immune-suppressing drugs opened the door to transplants. These images are from the first US heart transplant in 1967.

B   The 1960s saw extraordinary developments in heart surgery. Heart conditions such as atherosclerosis, where plaque builds up inside the arteries, were no longer death sentences. Here, the pioneering US surgeon Dr Michael DeBakey is at work.

Immune suppression Refers in this context to the deliberate and targeted medical suppression of the body's immune response to prevent the rejection of a transplanted organ. Diseases such as AIDS and lymphoma can also suppress our immune systems.

Neuroscience The scientific study of the nervous system. It is a multi-disciplinary field that seeks to understand the properties of neurons, neural circuits and their implications both for health and for human society and culture.

No longer the result of a discrete external agent or 'germ', these diseases, often resistant to treatment, are pathological responses to our environments and the lives we choose, or are compelled, to lead. For all the money we throw at medicine – about 10% of global GDP or 7.6 trillion US dollars in 2015 – the great medical leaps of the late 19th and early 20th centuries are faltering.

When the NHS was created in Britain in 1948, it was argued that once the major sources of our ill health were tackled – conceived at the time as being the major communicative diseases – the need for health services would decline. Globally, the opposite has been uniformly true.

Paradoxically, the healthier we have become, the more health and health care we demand, and the more anxious we grow. Added to this, cures for a host of diseases – schizophrenia, Alzheimer's, even the simple common cold and its vicious cousin influenza – seem remote. And early successes have unforeseen consequences.

Epigenetics The study of heritable changes in the expression of genes independent of any changes in the underlying DNA sequence. It looks at biological mechanisms for switching different genes on or off.

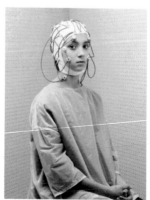
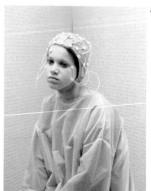

A

Greater knowledge has revealed greater complexity. For all the optimism that sequencing the human genome released, its therapeutic achievements have been scant. Few diseases are expressions of single genes; many of our most troubling and devastating conditions, such as depression, look more like the complex interaction of genes, environment, upbringing and luck. The new science of epigenetics has shown that environmental factors can trigger the expression of certain genes, and these changes can be heritable. We are more than the mechanical expression of our DNA. Is it time to temper some of our technological and prodigiously costly optimism?

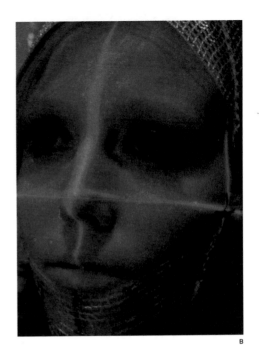

B

Waging war on pestilence wonderfully focused the medical mind, but today things are less certain. If longevity leads to senility, multiple morbidity and a catastrophic loss of independence, should the goal of medicine be to keep us alive at all costs, irrespective of the quality of our lives? Given the ballooning costs, the ceaseless proliferation of unintended consequences and the ever-present possibility of doing more harm than good, we need urgently to ask the question: what is the purpose of medicine today?

A Advances in neuroscience have made inroads into the final medical frontier: the human brain. Findings are tantalizing, but the possibility of direct medical intervention in the brain raises ethical questions.

B Few modern diseases provoke fear like cancer. Although longevity has improved for many, cancer remains a lethal killer. Here, crossed lasers accurately aim neutron beams in cancer treatment.

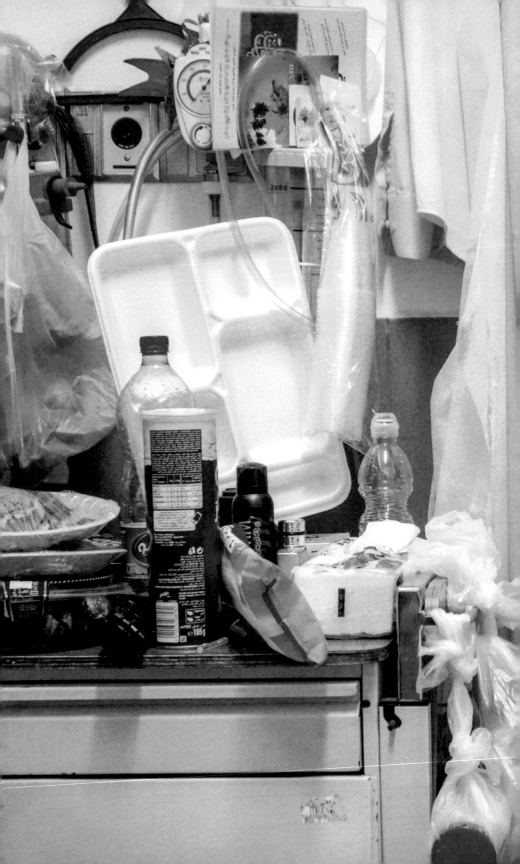

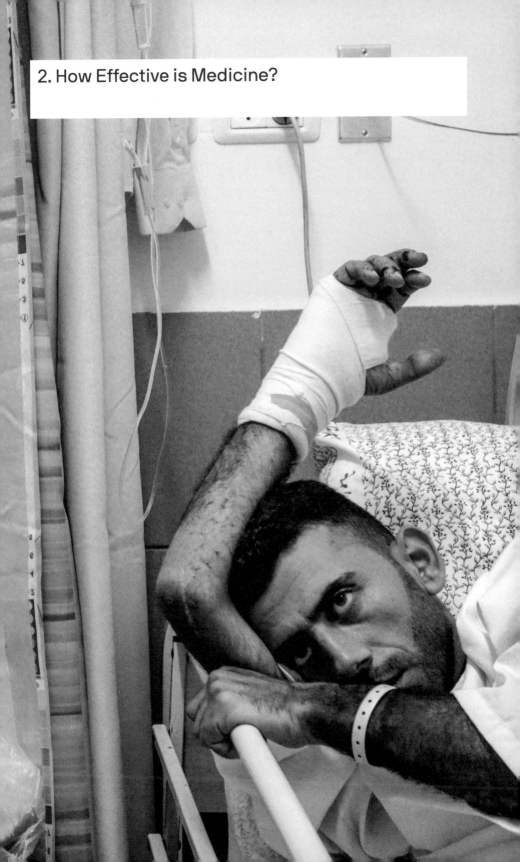

2. How Effective is Medicine?

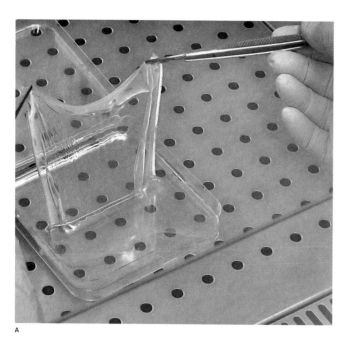

A

Palliative care Care provided to terminal patients for whom curative interventions are no longer indicated. It can include pain relief and emotional, psychological and spiritual support.

Opioids Drugs that act directly on the central nervous system and are usually used for the management of acute or chronic pain. They can create dependency and are fatal at overdose, so they are often controlled.

In 2015, doctors in Germany were preparing to transfer a dying young Syrian boy to palliative care. He was suffering from junctional epidermolysis bullosa, a rare genetic disease that leads to fragile and blistering skin. Apart from a small patch on his thigh, he had lost the entire surface of his skin. All available treatment had failed and he was on morphine to control pain. A team of Italian doctors tried an experimental genetic treatment. They took epidermal cells from the remaining patch of skin and used a virus to correct a defective gene called LAMB3. They grew colonies of the new cells in the laboratory, which developed into sheets of genetically modified skin – almost enough for his entire body. During two operations, they grafted them onto his body. Within a month, the graft had started to take. The new skin included stem cells, enabling the transplanted skin to renew and sustain itself. Two years on, the boy is at school and playing football. He needs no ointment or medication, and as the skin was made from his own cells, he does not need drugs to suppress rejection.

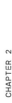

It is difficult not to be awestruck. Although genetic medicine has struggled to fulfil its early therapeutic hype, this is in the spirit of earlier heroic innovations: an individual life saved, hope for millions suffering with debilitating skin conditions.

But there is another side. Consider the slow-moving public health disaster unfolding in the USA. Drug overdoses, principally prescription opioids or their illegal substitutes, are now the primary cause of death in the under 50s in the USA.

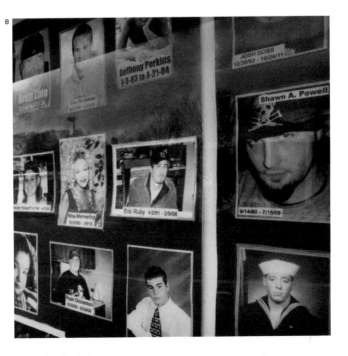

A   A genetically engineered sheet of skin is grown in the laboratory to treat a rare genetic disorder that leads to blistering skin. Modern genetic medicine holds out the hope of extraordinary developments in therapeutic techniques.

B   A memorial wall for victims of drug abuse and violence in Ohio. Despite huge technological advances in some areas of medicine, death from opioid addiction in the USA has reduced life expectancy in the world's wealthiest country.

In 2015, there were 142 fatal drug overdoses a day, 52,000 for the year, most of them involving opioid addiction. In 2016, the figure leapt to nearly 63,000, over 170 people a day, more than car accidents and shootings combined.

This is a complex story, with many players and multiple causes, but there is no doubt that medicine, in the form of prescriptions for highly addictive – and aggressively marketed – painkillers, had a big, early hand in it. The origins of the current opioid epidemic can almost certainly be traced to the mid 1990s when US drug companies promoted legal narcotics, particularly the slow-release, semi-synthetic opioid OxyContin. On the back of a sophisticated and extremely profitable marketing campaign, OxyContin was heavily promoted by doctors as a remedy for all kinds of pain. Patients were assured it was safe, but in fact it wasn't. Although prescribed in huge quantities, OxyContin is highly addictive. When the problem was finally acknowledged and distribution was restricted, people turned to black market fentanyl – with deadly results. By 2015, more than 2 million Americans were addicted to opioids, while 97.5 million – 36.4% of the population –used prescription painkillers.

Pain, both physical and psychological, is endemic in human life.

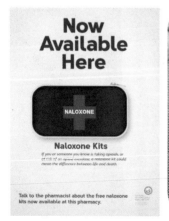

Now Available Here

NALOXONE

Naloxone Kits

If you or someone you know is taking opioids, or at risk of an opioid overdose, a naloxone kit could mean the difference between life and death.

Talk to the pharmacist about the free naloxone kits now available at this pharmacy.

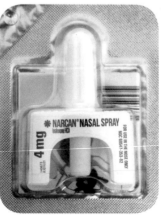

★ NARCAN® NASAL SPRAY

4 mg

A

Fentanyl
A powerful synthetic (laboratory-made) opioid, chemically similar to morphine but between 50 and 100 times more potent. It is a prescription-only drug used to manage severe pain, frequently post-operatively.

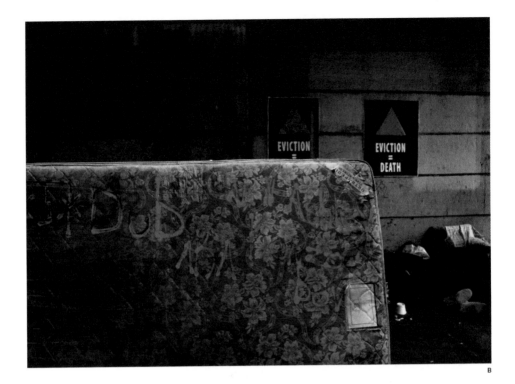

B

A   In 2018, the US Surgeon General issued a public health advisory to encourage more people to carry and learn to use Naloxone kits. The drug can be administered as an injection or a nasal spray (Narcan) and it suspends the effects of an opioid overdose until emergency responders arrive. There is, however, cause for concern regarding the increasing cost of Naloxone.

B   The opioid epidemic in the USA has hit the homeless, including those at this homeless encampment in Philadelphia. Poverty, ill health and systemic barriers to health services all take their toll.

Painkillers, for obvious reasons highly prized in human cultures, are not therapeutic: they do not treat the underlying problem or disorder; they palliate the pain symptoms. There is seldom a free lunch in nature.

Like most medical interventions, painkillers have unintended and often undesirable side effects; opioids are well known for their addictive qualities, for example. Good medicine will seek a positive balance between the benefits and harms of an intervention.

Medicine is a complex field of human activity and experience – asking how effective it is can be challenging.

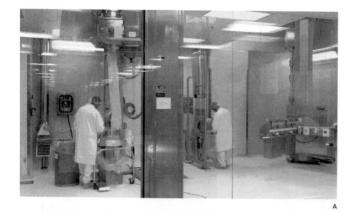

A Pharmaceuticals is a major global industry. Every medicinal benefit has a side effect, and these side effects are a major source of global morbidity and mortality. Here, workers are checking pharmaceutical products at an Israeli manufacturer.

B Consumer expectations – of permanent, pain-free health, and a quick medical fix – can lead directly to the prescription pad. For drug companies and for commercial health providers, meeting these expectations means big business. This huge depot is a pharmaceutical distribution centre in Antwerp, Belgium.

C Medicine and health care are highly politicized. In the USA, the political wrestle over Obamacare and attempts to make access to health care more democratic reveal the political issues at stake. Powerful commercial interests support private medicine. Republicans are seen in action here at their convention in Ohio in 2016.

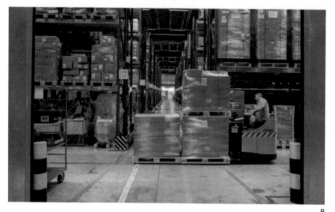

B

Some treatments are highly effective for some people some of the time. Some things that are effective for one person will be ineffective, or actively toxic, for another. But the US opioid crisis reveals several factors pushing medicine in a dangerous direction.

Some of these, like poor prescription practices, are internal to medicine and amenable to fixes from within. Others are not. Take patient expectation. Partly because of medicine's success and partly due to social expectations of endlessly increasing happiness, people turn to medicine to free themselves from suffering, almost irrespective of its nature or origin.

Powerful corporations, particularly pharmaceutical companies, recognize the huge profits that lie in meeting these expectations. Doctors understandably want to relieve the suffering of their patients. In private, fee-for-service medicine, this can be lucrative and serious conflicts of interest arise. If a patient wants a powerful painkiller, and a doctor will be paid for its provision, the inclination to prescribe is clear. Pressure on doctors' time, combined with patients' desire for treatment, can have a similar effect.

A doctor who suggests a conservative approach, a stoic acceptance that life is not pain-free and warns that the medicine may, in time, be worse than the illness, is swimming against the tide.

For all the horrors of opioid addiction, a far more troubling global medical disaster is looming: antibiotic resistance.

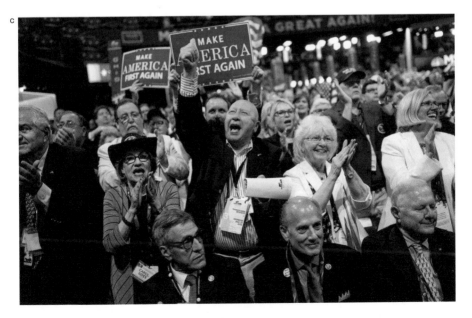

c

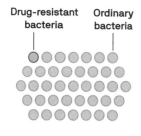

Drug-resistant bacteria | Ordinary bacteria

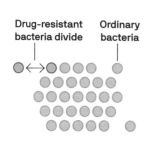

Drug-resistant bacteria divide | Ordinary bacteria

Drug-resistant bacteria continue to multiply

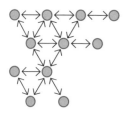

Drug-resistant bacteria

A

In part, this is a natural process, the outcome of an unceasing Darwinian struggle between bacteria and the antibiotics that target them. Bacteria randomly mutate in nature, and some of these mutations confer immunity; some bacteria also acquire immunity from others. But widespread misuse, including over-prescription, their massive use in livestock and problems with patient adherence to drug regimes, is accelerating the process. Superbugs such as MRSA, or multi-drug resistant microbes are emerging, which put hospital patients at risk of a serious, hard-to-treat infection.

A As living organisms with a terrifyingly fast reproduction rate, bacteria can rapidly develop immunity to antibiotics. This natural process is exacerbated by the misuse of antibiotics. Diseases we once thought almost eradicated are returning.

B Drug-resistant tuberculosis is threatening a global health tragedy as a Victorian killer mutates. In the dish on the left, bacteria will not develop near the antibiotics. On the right, antibiotic-resistant bacteria are growing.

Tragically, we are seeing the return of a disease thought confined to the history of Victorian sanatoria: tuberculosis (TB). Partly again, this is natural selection: survival selects those strains of bacteria that do not succumb to antibiotics, and they multiply. But it is also the result of poor treatment and lack of patient adherence to drug regimens: treatment for TB can be lengthy and toxic. Strains of TB resistant to first-line treatments – known as multi-drug resistant TB (MDR-TB) – are emerging. More worrying are strains resistant to second-line treatments, known as extremely drug-resistant TB (XDR-TB).

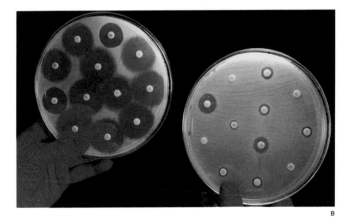

B

MRSA (methicillin-resistant Staphylococcus aureus) A type of bacteria, sometimes referred to as a 'superbug', that is resistant to many first-line antibiotics and can therefore be difficult to treat. Although it can live naturally and harmlessly on the skin, it can be dangerous for those with pre-existing illnesses.

Market failure A term used in economics to refer to a set of circumstances where the allocation of resources in a free market is inefficient. This includes circumstances where the quantity of goods required by customers is not the same as the quantity produced by suppliers.

The antibiotic crisis is also a potentially devastating example of market failure in medicine. Most pharmaceutical companies no longer undertake antibiotic research, and only two new classes of antibiotics have been introduced in the past 40 years.

Unlike statins, which patients usually take for life and hence provide a long-term return on investment, antibiotics are given for short periods. As they are a response to immediately life-threatening conditions, prices are often forced down. And because they are vulnerable to resistance, their shelf life can be short. It is simply not economically viable for pharmaceutical companies to invest.

When assessing how effective medicine is, it is also worth looking at the day to day, nuts and bolts of medicine and the ineradicable presence of uncertainty. Few people not practising medicine are aware of just how uncertain it is, for all its claims to science. Consider interventions for two common conditions: prostate cancer and back pain.

Prostate cancer is the most common cancer among men. Globally, in 2012, more than 1.1 million cases were recorded: about 15% of new cancers in men. Rates were highest in Martinique, followed by Norway and France. There are approximately 10,000 deaths in Britain a year, closer to 30,000 in the USA.

Prostate cancer is usually identified by an initial prostate-specific antigen blood test, with confirmation via biopsy. Where cancer is identified, several responses are offered: monitoring or watchful waiting without active therapy, surgical removal of the prostate (prostatectomy), hormone therapy or some form of radiotherapy. Sometimes several treatments are combined. The difficulty is identifying which forms are life-threatening. Many men die *with* rather than *of* prostate cancer, and there is currently no reliable way to distinguish between aggressive and indolent tumours. Both radiotherapy and prostatectomy have potentially serious side effects, including bowel problems, incontinence and impotence. (It is partly for fear of over-treatment that many countries avoid routine population screening for prostate cancer.) Doctors and patients are therefore in a difficult position. Identifying prostate cancer is relatively straightforward, if not, in the case of biopsy, pain- or risk-free. Yet having identified it, there is real uncertainty about treatment. For many, a diagnosis of cancer is terrifying, and they will opt for radical treatment to remove it. However, in many but not all cases, this means unnecessary treatment with unpleasant and enduring side effects.

Most decisions about treatment are made in the face of uncertainty.

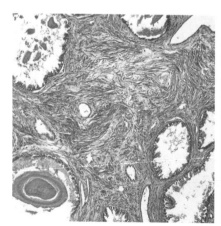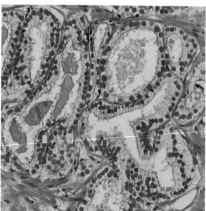

A

A Although a major killer, prostate cancer – depicted here in a light micrograph – presents treatment problems for doctors and patients. It is still not possible to identify which prostate cancers are life-threatening. Given the serious side effects of treatment, uncertainty remains about the best course of action.

B Although our expectations of modern medicine are ever-increasing – and the technology designed to meet those expectations is ever more expensive – returns are diminishing. Many of those treated for prostate cancer, including those treated, as here, by external beam radiotherapy, may not have benefited.

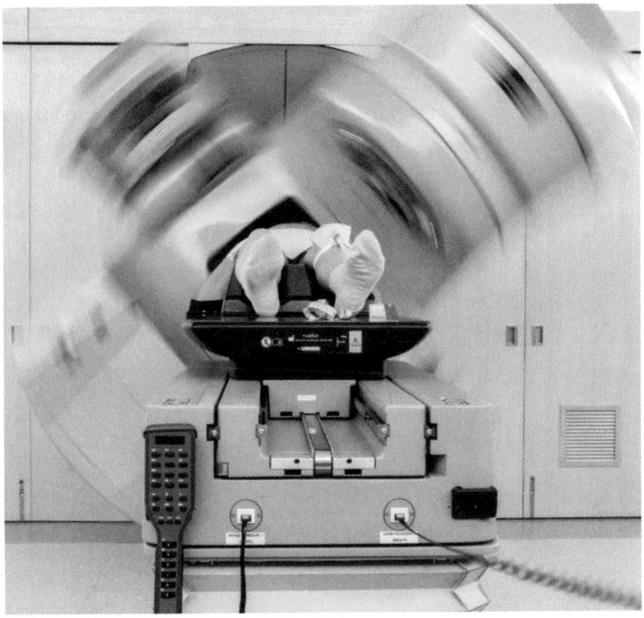

B

Population screening The systematic testing of a specific, usually asymptomatic, population for a discrete disorder to identify those who require either direct treatment or further investigation.

MRI scan A type of scan that uses powerful magnetic forces and radio waves to produce detailed images of the inside of the body. Unlike X-rays, it does not use ionizing radiation and consequently has much lower risk.

Now consider the use of MRI scans (magnetic resonance imaging) for back pain. Back pain is among the largest causes of disability in the world. Although MRI scans are almost entirely risk-free and provide a wonderfully detailed and intimate image of the spine, they are expensive, time-consuming and, in many if not most cases of back pain, almost entirely useless. Most back pain is non-specific, which is a polite way of saying that nobody knows where it comes from. And this is where scans can be unhelpful. The spine is subject to natural wear and tear. As we age, our spine changes, just as our skin loses its elasticity and our hair its colour and shine. An MRI scan of the spine is likely to reveal these changes, but it cannot indicate if they are the source of the pain. A research study of MRI scans performed on healthy people with no back pain found abnormalities in 87% of scans.

The problem is not reserved for back pain and spinal scans. Our bodies are imperfect and they change with ageing. Recent years have seen the proliferation of commercial, direct-to-customer diagnostic testing – anything from DNA sequencing to identify risk factors, to brain scans to detect pre-malignant changes in brain structure. But little of this information can identify clinically significant changes. Without professional expertise to interpret the findings, it can lead to anxiety; nothing provokes worry among the well better than 'scientific' proof of abnormalities, or apparently menacing shadows and shapes on a brilliant MRI scan. In addition to anxiety, it can lead to further expensive and unnecessary diagnostic tests. In turn, these may result in unnecessary treatment with the risk of side effects.

As we will see in Chapter 3, it is not only uncertainty and anxiety driving over-diagnosis and over-treatment. Disease definitions are being expanded and diagnostic thresholds lowered. More people are identified as being in pre-disease or pre-morbid states and are targeted for early interventions. This can be a good thing. Potentially life-threatening conditions can be identified while treatable. But it can also lead to the identification of conditions in people that will not develop symptoms and that will certainly not kill them. And over-diagnosis can be harmful. It can label healthy people as ill, expose them to the harms of unnecessary treatment and waste health resources better spent elsewhere.

A

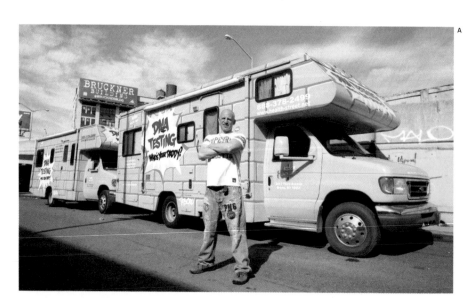

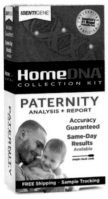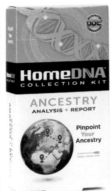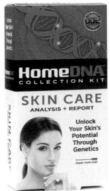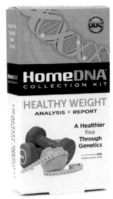

B

Increased medical activity with no health gain is the definition of too much medicine.

A classic case of over-diagnosis and over-treatment is thyroid cancer. In a deft research article from 2013, US health care researcher Juan Brito and colleagues showed how the use of increasingly sophisticated diagnostic techniques led to a threefold increase in the detection of papillary thyroid cancer in the past 30 years, with absolutely no corresponding change in mortality.

DNA sequencing The identification of the precise order of the four chemical building blocks in a DNA molecule. Provides information about the genetic information carried in a particular strand or segment of DNA.

A Entrepreneur Jared Rosenthal set up a mobile DNA testing van in 2010. The explosion in direct-to-customer diagnostics means we can find out more about our underlying health state. How much of this information can be translated into meaningful clinical findings is less certain.

B It is possible that the information disclosed by these home DNA testing kits would need careful medical interpretation and explanation. More information is not always better. Testing can lead to over-diagnosis and costly, unnecessary treatment.

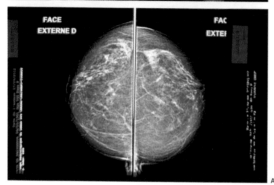

FACE EXTERNE D

FAC EXTE

A

Commercial players such as drug companies and manufacturers of medical devices have a strong interest in expanding disease categories. In 2014, Australian health journalist Ray Moynihan and colleagues studied 16 publications from national and international guideline panels defining diagnostic criteria for 12 common conditions in the USA. Out of 16 published between 2000 and 2013, ten widened the definition, one restricted it and in five the impact was uncertain. An average of 75% of panel members had ties to industry and twelve of the panels were chaired by people with corporate links.

Population screening can also drive over-diagnosis and unnecessary treatment. Screening involves the systematic testing of a defined and usually asymptomatic population for a specific disorder. It can identify people at risk of serious diseases, such as cancer, who are not yet symptomatic. But there are downsides. Screening tests are not invariably accurate; they can give both false positive and negative results and can lead to the labelling of healthy people as sick. They can also trigger over-treatment in those who would never have gone on to develop clinically significant illness.

In recent decades, medicine has responded to uncertainty by making strong claims for evidence-based medicine. Evidence generated from randomized controlled trials (RCTs) should replace the almost folkloric reliance on tradition and theoretically informed intuition – historical mainstays of clinical medicine.

There have been successes: evidence-based guidelines led to significant improvement in asthma care and the prevention of post-surgical embolism. But RCTs often focus on single disorders, excluding those with complex co-morbidities. In real life, co-morbidities are commonplace, so how useful are RCTs to clinical practice? Over-zealous application of guidelines can mean clinicians end up treating statistical averages rather than individual patients. Drug companies often set research agendas, and conflicts of interest among the developers of evidence-based guidelines are widespread. More unsettling still, as Stanford professor John Ioannidis demonstrated in a paper published in 2005, there are good reasons to believe that a great deal of published research is unreliable.

A Routine breast screening
– carried out here by
mammography – can lead to the
identification of early cancers.
However, it can give rise to
false positives and negatives,
labelling healthy people sick.
B A Russian patient trials a drug
for osteoporosis. Randomized
control trials are the mainstay
of evidence-based medicine,
but their focus on single
disorders raises questions about
the applicability of results.

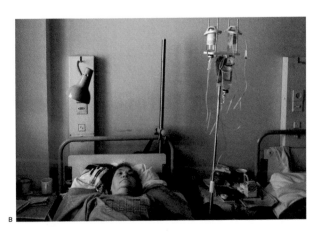

B

McDonald's Original size Coke

7-11 Big Gulp

7-11 Team Gulp

McDonald's Supersize

Kum & Go's HuMUGous

McDonald's kid-sized soda

KFC Mega Jug

2006

McDonald's largest soda

2011

2005

1980

1999

128 oz

1974

100 oz

2018

64 oz

1955

32 oz

42 oz

7 oz

12 oz

21 oz

A

A bitter irony of modern life is that having vanquished so many threats to our health, the diseases of affluence are now killing us. Consider obesity. According to the World Health Organization (WHO), one in three of the world's adult population is overweight and one in ten obese. And the health consequences of obesity are stark. They include cardiovascular disease, stroke, hypertension, depression, musculo-skeletal disorders such as osteoarthritis, type 2 diabetes and several cancers, including breast, colon, kidney, liver and endometrial. At the same time, nearly 800 million globally suffer from calorie deficiency and 2 billion from micronutrient malnutrition. It is possible to be obese and malnourished.

Obesity, like other diseases of lifestyle, reveals the limits of medicine. Aside from advising about lifestyle changes, medical practitioners are restricted to imperfect patch jobs on the body's pathological responses to extreme weight gain and the effects of alcohol, drugs or tobacco. Of 74 interventions designed to tackle obesity identified by the McKinsey Global Institute in 2014, only four involved direct therapy. Tackling the diseases of lifestyle involves taking on both private choices and the underlying social architecture behind them. The role of medicine is modest.

No branch of medicine is more contested, controversial and uncertain than psychiatry.

Thomas Szasz (1920–2012), former professor of psychiatry at Syracuse University in New York, famously, controversially, decreed mental illness a myth. For Szasz, a body can be diseased, but not a mind. Talk of mental illness is metaphorical, the transfer of categories belonging to physical medicine to the human psyche and human behaviour. And the process is not benign. The 'medicalization' of mental suffering – the 'manufacture of madness' – serves both the professional interests of psychiatry and social needs for regimentation and control. Outside of psychiatry, the French historian and philosopher Michel Foucault (1926–84) argued that the objective 'science' of mental illness was nothing of the sort. It had nothing to do with health but was a surreptitious method for imposing social control on those who sought to live differently.

These ideas, associated with the anti-psychiatry movement of the 1960s and 1970s, do not seem as urgent today. Partly, this stems from social and institutional change. In the West, the era of the huge psychiatric asylums is over. Today, you are more likely to hear of the struggle to get appropriate psychiatric support for the most seriously mentally ill. Those with serious mental disorders can be horrifically vulnerable. Championing their liberty can seem a betrayal of their needs for care and support.

Micronutrient malnutrition A dietary lack or deficiency of essential vitamins or minerals. Often used to refer to diseases caused by such a deficiency, such as anaemia and pellagra. It has been estimated that more than 2 billion people may be affected by micronutrient malnutrition globally.

Anti-psychiatry A loose political and social movement with its origins in the 1960s, characterized by the view that psychiatry is not a science but a coercive form of social control more likely to result in harm to individuals than therapeutic benefit. Associated with the work of the sociologist RD Laing in Britain and Thomas Szasz in the USA.

B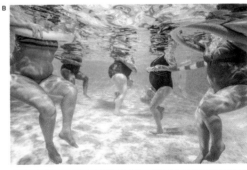
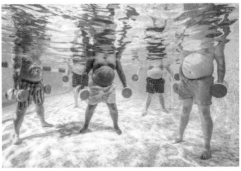

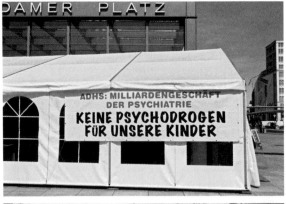

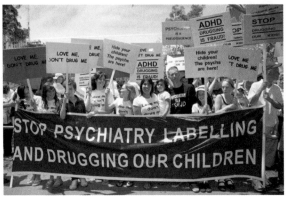

A

Selective serotonin reuptake inhibitors (SSRIs) The most widely prescribed family of anti-depressants in the world, SSRIs boost levels of serotonin in the brain. Serotonin has a variety of functions, including as a neurotransmitter. Largely found in the human gut, it is associated with mood regulation.

Diagnostic and Statistical Manual of Mental Disorders (DSM) Published by the American Psychiatric Association, the manual aims to provide objective criteria for the diagnosis of mental disorders. The most recent version (DSM 5) was met with some controversy as to the objective existence of some of the disorders listed.

Even in its heyday, anti-psychiatry had to contend with the reality of mental suffering and the evidence that the symptoms of many psychiatric conditions were stable over time, suggesting a real rather than metaphysical disease.

The use of lithium to stabilize bipolar disorder, the rise of neuroscience, the possibilities suggested by neuro-imaging, the identification of associations between certain genes and mental illness, and the early optimism associated with the new generation of selective serotonin reuptake inhibitors (SSRIs) to treat depression have tilted opinion against the social construction of mental illness.

But problems remain. Mental health conditions are more easily influenced by social norms than physical ones.

It was not until 1973 that homosexuality was removed from the US psychiatry bible, the *Diagnostic and Statistical Manual of Mental Disorders* (DSM). You do not have to go back in time far to find absurdity: in 1851, the US physician Samuel Cartwright (1793–1863) published a paper proposing a new mental disorder: drapetomania – the desire of slaves to run away.

In 2013, the publication of the new DSM 5 reignited the debate about whether psychiatric conditions point to disease entities. Disease thresholds were lowered, new diseases – internet addiction, shyness in children, skin-picking disorder – were added. In Britain, the Division of Clinical Psychology of the British Psychological Society rubbished the entire enterprise – such diagnoses, it argued, 'were of limited reliability and questionable validity'.

Consider depression, now vying with musculo-skeletal problems as the leading cause of disability globally. Where is the sufferer to turn? One highly articulate sufferer of severe depression was William Styron (1925–2006), author of *Sophie's Choice* (1979).

A   Psychiatry attends to human behaviour and thought, as well as brain chemistry. It remains vulnerable to criticism for enforcing social norms rather than treating disease. Supporters of anti-psychiatry are seen here protesting against children being medicated.

B   Patients at a hospital in Hefei, China, line up to receive medicine from nurses. The hospital accepts about 100 patients who are suffering from mental illness. Only 10% of the 30 million Chinese currently suffering from depression receive proper medical care.

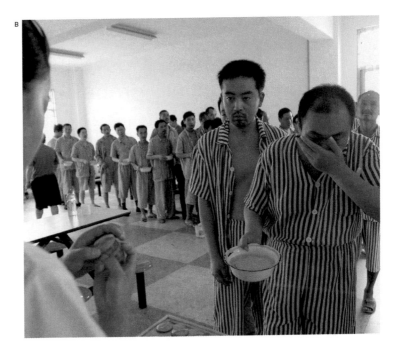

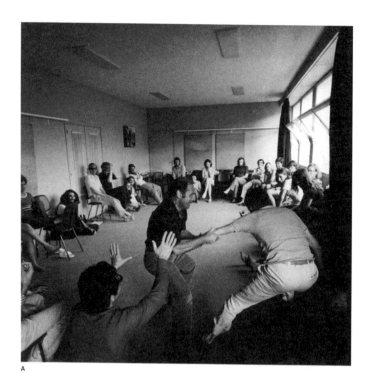

A

Surveying the field at the end of the 1980s, he wrote: 'The intense and sometimes comically strident factionalism that exists in present-day psychiatry – the schism between the believers in psychotherapy and the adherents of pharmacology – resembles the medical quarrels of the 18th century (to bleed or not to bleed) and almost defines . . . the inexplicable nature of depression and its treatment.'

Fast forward 25 years, and where are we? Most sufferers of depression will probably be offered antidepressants. A 2017 update from the US National Library of Medicine suggests that between 40 and 60% of people taking an antidepressant improved. But then so did between 20 and 40% of those taking a placebo. Research suggests that overall, about one-third of sufferers will benefit from antidepressants.

Evidence also suggests that cognitive behaviour therapy is as effective as medication, and that further improvements are achieved by combining the two. But if drugs that address serotonin levels in our brains are as effective – but not necessarily more effective – than a chemical-free therapy designed to interrupt the negative cycle of thought and mood reinforcement, where are we with our understanding of the leading mental disorder of our times? Are we further than one of Styron's psychiatrists who said: 'If you compare our knowledge with Columbus' discovery of America, America is yet unknown; we are still down on that little island in the Bahamas.'?

The tension between the expectations of modern medicine and the reality of human vulnerability is clearest in the medicalization of death.

Speculative futurology notwithstanding, it is reasonable to assume that we are mortal – that our bodies wear out and, sooner or later, we die.

To defer death and ease our suffering, we turn to medicine. And with good reason.

Take life expectancy. Although not exclusively attributable to clinical medicine, the achievement is stunning. According to *The Economist,* the average lifespan increased more over the past four generations than in the previous 8,000. In 1900, global life expectancy was about 32 years. It is now 71.8. Much of this is due to lower child and infant mortality, but not all of it. Someone who was 60 years old in 2011 would be expected to live until they are 85. And not only have we deferred death, advances in pain control have made dying, in most cases, less painful – although probably not less frightening.

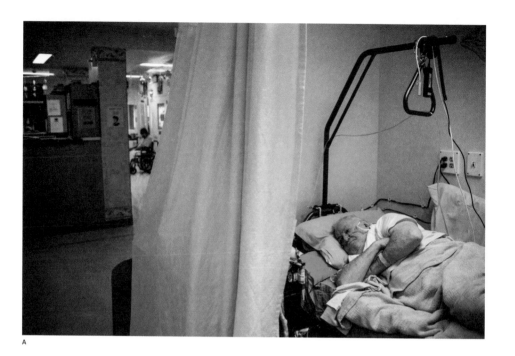

A

These achievements have a downside. Death ceases to be a natural terminus and becomes a medical event – and given medicine's purpose, a failure.

Increasingly, we die anything but a natural or peaceful death. We die in intensive treatment units, plugged into banks of machinery. Or we die in nursing homes, among strangers. Is this good medicine? Are we prolonging life or brutally extending our dying?

In hospital, the weeks before death are often filled with frenetic medical activity, much of it pointless. For the past 20 years, research has been telling us that 'non-beneficial treatment' is widespread at the end of life. There are many reasons: the difficulty of predicting death with accuracy, varieties of defensive practice – from fear of litigation to doctors' reluctance to have patients die on their watch – and the desire to show relatives that everything possible has been done. (More than one in ten Americans with terminal cancer have chemotherapy in their last fortnight, despite it conferring no benefit; 8% have surgery in their last week.) Is this how we want to spend the last days of our lives?

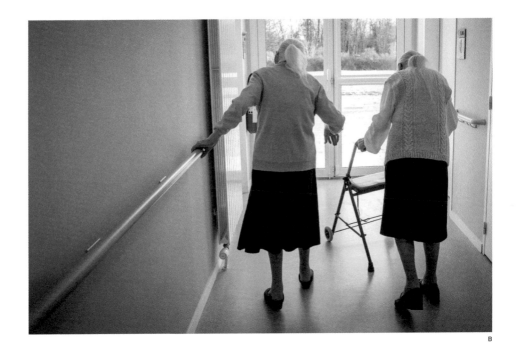

This intense focus on high-tech therapeutic intervention, with its subliminal refusal to accept the inevitability of death, can lead to the neglect of good palliative care. Where death is accepted as inevitable, attention can turn to easing the patient's passage and ensuring they can make the best use of remaining time. Currently, end of life care risks becoming a futile high-tech assault on the inevitable. And nobody but the manufacturers and pay-for-service providers seem to benefit. Is this really where we want to invest so much of our medical resources?

Medicine can be effective, sometimes spectacularly so. But as the medicalization of death makes clear, more medicine is not always more effective. Sometimes it is harmful: the gains marginal, the burdens considerable. As we will see in Chapter 3, there are significant pressures driving the expansion of medicine into more and more areas of human experience.

Is life solely a medical phenomenon?

A   Jim Robelen, a hospice patient diagnosed with terminal pulmonary fibrosis, is cared for at the California Medical Facility. Created in 1991, it is the first prison hospice programme.

B   Centenary twins Paulette Olivier and Simone Thiot at a retirement home in 2016. They are believed to be the oldest twins in the world.

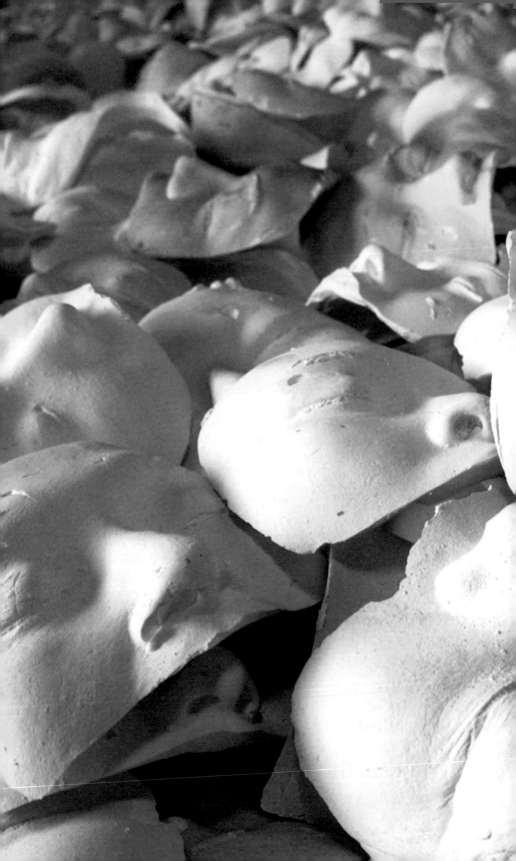

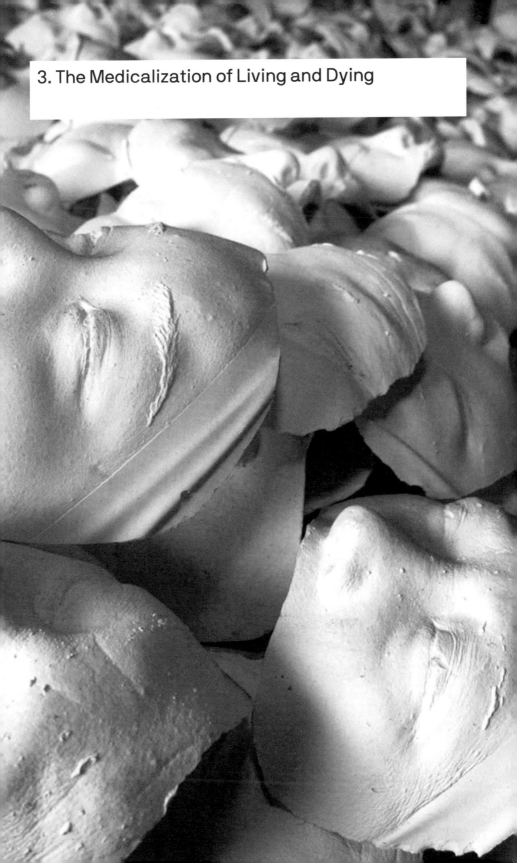

3. The Medicalization of Living and Dying

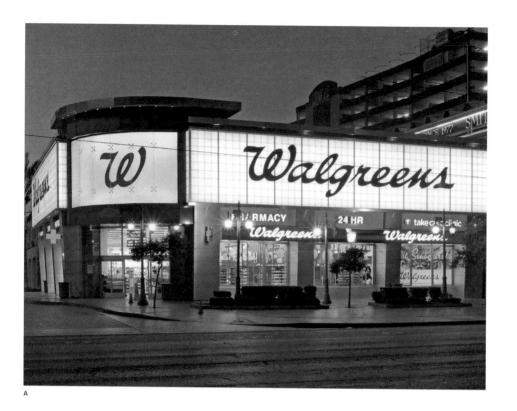

A

What do we mean by a medical problem? What aspects of our experience, of our functioning and dysfunctioning, are the proper object of medical concern? Put more simply, when and about what should we make an appointment with our doctor?

There may have been a time when the answer was obvious. During those long millennia when medicine was impotent, medical problems

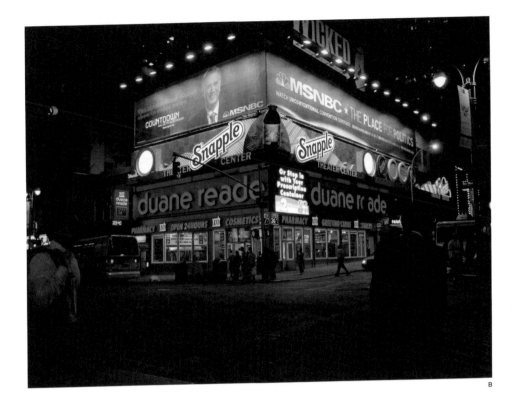

were those that threatened to kill our bodies or unsettle our minds. For everything else there was a priest, a herbalist and whatever capacity we had to endure.

But medicine has become more successful and our knowledge of human functioning has expanded. We want to be rid of more and more impediments to our well-being.

The commercial purveyors of medicine and its goods and services push to expand their markets and so the scope of medical interest has widened.

A   Opening its first store in Chicago in 1901, Walgreens is now part of the largest retail pharmacy group in the US and Europe.
B   New York's favourite drug store, Duane Reade. Americans are among the biggest prescription drug users in the world.

The name given to this process is medicalization. Sociologists first identified it in the 1960s. Their focus was the medicalization of 'deviance' – declaring anti-social behaviour a medical or biological rather than a social or normative problem – but the term was relevant to the way human experience increasingly fell under medical scrutiny. Put simply, medicalization is the process by which human conditions come to be medical problems. Examples include childbirth, attention deficit hyperactivity disorder (ADHD) in children, alcoholism, menopause, erectile dysfunction in older men, ageing, infertility, grieving, obesity, baldness and death itself. Medicalization also extends to behaviours. Child abuse, domestic violence, gambling and promiscuity – sex addiction – have all become subjects of medical interest.

Early writings on medicalization were critical. In his classic *Medical Nemesis* (1975), the Austrian philosopher Ivan Illich (1926–2002) thunderously denounced the industrialized medicalization of modern society. 'Once a society is so organized that medicine can transform people into patients because they are unborn, newborn, menopausal or at some other 'age of risk', the population inevitably loses some of its autonomy to its healers.' *Medical Nemesis* is still a bracing and necessary read, but it has aged. Currently, medicalization is regarded as the outcome of a far more complex set of processes.

Medicalization The complex process, or set of processes, by which more and more areas of human life and experience come to be regarded as medical issues and therefore require medical intervention. It is often associated with the redefinition of 'ordinary' human experience as illness or disorder, opening the way to medical treatment.

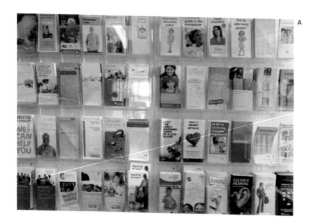

A

Attention deficit hyperactivity disorder (ADHD) A behavioural disorder, usually associated with onset in early childhood, with symptoms including inattentiveness, hyperactivity and impulsiveness. Although the symptoms tend to ease with adulthood, some adults experience ongoing problems.

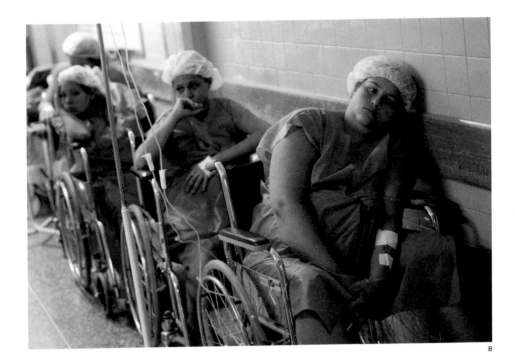

B

Today, medicalization is multi-dimensional. The medical profession remains important, although it can both increase medicalization and – as a gatekeeper for access to publicly funded medical services – struggle to contain it. But other actors are significant. Social movements, including patient groups, can seek a medical construction – a 'diagnosis' – for a disorder. A medical diagnosis can confer legitimacy and counter stigma, particularly where there are suggestions that the condition is 'all in the mind'. (Although there is evidence that ascribing biological causes to mental illnesses increases stigma.) Social support, such as disability allowance, specialist educational facilities or changes to the work-place, requires medical certification. Health insurance requires diagnosis to trigger payment.

A   There are few areas of human experience in which modern medicine does not take an interest, as this plethora of leaflets on display in a doctor's surgery shows. More and more of us turn to doctors for relief from problems that are only questionably 'medical'.

B   Pregnant women await a C-section. The medicalization of childbirth has brought enormous benefits. Disagreement persists though about the extent of medical involvement, with some extolling the virtues of home birth, while others seek surgical intervention.

Consider in this context the extraordinary journey of the central nervous stimulant methylphenidate, better known by the trade name Ritalin. Before focusing on the compound though, we need to look at the condition it primarily addresses: ADHD. As with so many of the issues here, we are stepping straight into controversy.

Evidence from brain imaging suggests that those with ADHD have differences in their pre-frontal cortexes. Research also suggests a hereditary component. People diagnosed with ADHD respond well to therapy, but clinical disagreement remains. Some doctors, while recognizing the reality of the problem, do not believe the condition exists. They argue that ADHD refers to a set of behaviours. In most cases, methylphenidate is effective in managing them, although it has side effects: it can restrict growth and suppress appetite. However, it does not necessarily follow that there is a discrete condition – a disease entity – that lies behind the behaviours and causes them. The label ADHD is attached to the behaviours.

Ritalin The most commonly known brand name for the central nervous system stimulant methylphenidate. It is used principally as a treatment for ADHD but also for narcolepsy. Principal benefits include improving and maintaining alertness.

Whether or not there is a disease entity, diagnoses of ADHD have leapt. In the USA, it is now the second most frequent childhood diagnosis, just behind asthma. Between 2004

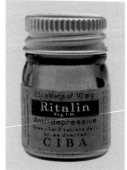
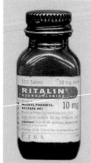
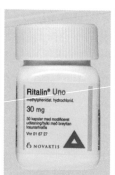
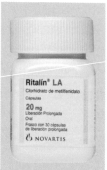

A

A The use of Ritalin, a stimulant for the central nervous system, has rocketed in recent years. Initially used for the treatment of ADHD, mainly among schoolchildren, it has increasingly become a lifestyle drug for those seeking to enhance their mental performance.

B Although there is some evidence from MRI scans of the brain – seen here – that those with ADHD have changes in their pre-frontal cortexes, the existence of ADHD as a discrete disease condition – rather than the description of a set of behaviours – is contested.

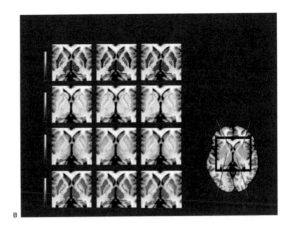

B

and 2014, diagnosed cases in Britain doubled; in 2014, they were approaching 1 million. Many argue that this is because of increasing awareness of the condition. Critics argue that we are at risk of medicalizing ordinary human behaviour, particularly among boys. Are we treating a medical condition or medicalizing behaviour that teachers and parents find difficult? Controversy continues.

There is no doubt that sales of methylphenidate are stratospheric. This is because it works. Children respond rapidly: their focus and attention increase, impulse control improves, disruptive behaviour dwindles.

But its effectiveness is not limited to children. Adults, particularly in the USA, are being diagnosed with ADHD. Increasingly, they are self-diagnosing, recognizing unwelcome aspects of their own behaviour or personality in its symptoms and seeking a diagnosis and medication to iron them out.

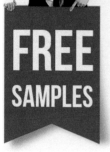
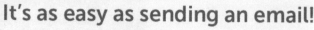
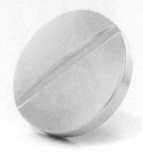
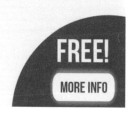
And what is true for those who see themselves, or are seen by others, as having a deficit in cognitive abilities is true for those who see themselves as normal but seek improvement. Methylphenidate can increase memory and attention among the healthy. Modanafil, ordinarily prescribed for sleep disorders, is said to give a 10% boost in cognitive powers, including memory, planning and impulse control. Along with other cognitive enhancers, these drugs are increasingly bought over the internet. Students use them for intense periods of study or while taking exams, with the aim of boosting their performance and, hopefully, their grades.

Cognitive enhancers Refers to drugs taken for the pharmaceutically driven improvement of aspects of human mental functioning, including memory, intelligence, concentration and cognition more widely.

Use of cognitive enhancers gives rise to ethical problems. Side effects notwithstanding, performance enhancers are banned in professional and Olympic sport. They are cheating. The purpose of the Olympics is to identify the finest athlete, not the best laboratory. Yet the use of cognitive enhancement does not give rise to the same qualms. But it is not obvious why they don't; after all, they also confer an advantage. If some people use them, the pressure on others to do the same increases. And if the purpose of study is academic excellence, and drugs can safely deliver it, shouldn't we be obliged to take them? Why settle for less rather than more of the excellence, whatever it is, that we pursue?

A Intelligence is among the most valuable – and marketable – human attributes, particularly in the hyper-competitive modern workplace. Little wonder that any drug seen to confer cognitive benefits, such as Modanafil, is a potential money-spinner.

B Medicinal drugs – or those derived from them – can be used to boost physical performance. Even the slightest advantage can be critical in ultra-competitive modern sports. Consequently, anti-doping controls are an essential component of Olympic and commercial sport.

Such ethical problems point to the potential scope of medicalization. Although the medical profession can be a sceptical and reluctant participant, the use of medical interventions to improve normal functioning suggests there is, in principle, no dimension of human functioning that cannot be medicalized. Where there is a market, and a product to meet it, there is no limit to its spread.

Medicalization is by no means always bad.

The expansion of medical interest in pregnancy and childbirth brought enormous benefits, slashing infant and maternal mortality rates. Globally, the World Health Organization estimates that infant mortality rates have declined from 64.8 deaths per 1,000 live births in 1990 to 30.5 in 2016. In the same period, maternal mortality rates declined by 44% – from 385 to 216 per 100,000 births.

B

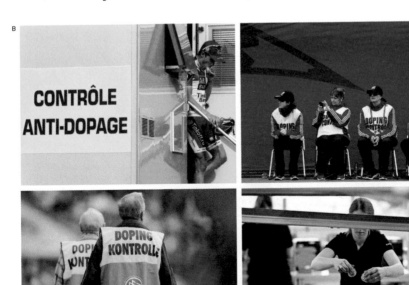

Not all of this has to do with medical involvement – and disputes remain about the scope of the medicalization of pregnancy and childbirth – but medicine has undoubtedly contributed. Similarly, the medicalization of human reproduction – the development of the contraceptive pill, the availability of abortion – has enormously increased women's ability to control reproductive choices.

Medicalization raises the question of whether medicine has a proper or appropriate field of study, such that anything within is properly medicalized and anything outside is not. It is tempting to say that the study of specific pathogens or diseases – the filoviruses, or cancer and diabetes – is properly medical while 'ordinary' or 'natural' unhappiness is not. Medicine, that is, should focus on properly 'organic' disorders: those with identifiable lesions or biomarkers.

However, scientific developments are undermining this distinction. Scientists increasingly see illness as a stage, or several stages, on a spectrum of variation. The idea of a distinction between diseased states – the proper focus of medical

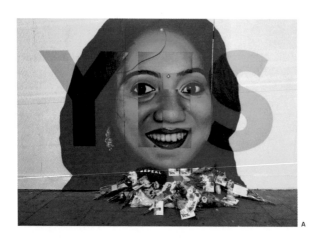

A The availability of contraception and safe abortion has increased women's reproductive rights. Here, flowers are left at a mural of Savita Halappanavar during the referendum on liberalizing abortion laws in Ireland in 2018. She died in 2012 after being denied an emergency termination.

B Modern medicine has a vital role to play in tackling emergent infectious diseases. Health care workers are seen here (left) at an Ebola treatment centre in Coyah, Guinea, in 2015. Disinfected gloves and boots (right) are hung out to dry.

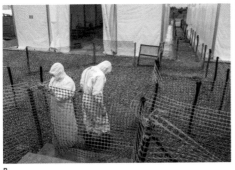
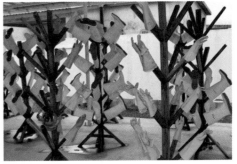

B

attention – and 'normal' or 'natural' states is retreating. We can no longer rely on nature to indicate what is or is not a disease. Increasingly, we have to decide for ourselves.

Although this can be a powerful tool for tackling stigma, it can open the door to medicalizing more of our experience. We may not be desperately sick, we may be asymptomatic, but this does not mean we are not on the spectrum. The scope of medical interest, and the size of the potential medical market, expands.

But is this necessarily a problem? If the medicalization of childbirth brought great benefits, why not target all human suffering, irrespective of its cause? If we are in pain and medicine can help, why worry if the complaint is narrowly medical? If a drug can remove some of the sting from extreme, although entirely natural, sadness, why not take it?

One practical reason, as with the opiate crisis in the USA, is that drugs have side effects, and some drugs have terrible side effects. Extreme grief is often protracted, and dependence upon pain relief must be a risk.

Filovirus Any member of the Filoviridae family of viruses, named after their filament-like structure. They cause haemorrhagic (related to bleeding or abnormal blood flow) fevers and include the viruses that cause Ebola and Marburg fevers.

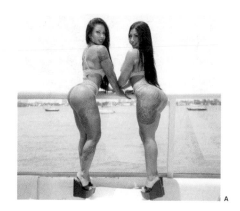
A

But what if we find a drug that has no, or only trivial, side effects? Why not use it?

Although we are approaching paradox, some pain may be good for us, even necessary. For all our technological brilliance, we are surprisingly vulnerable. Some experience of pain may strengthen us, simply because it may give us resources to manage it better when it next comes. A great deal of suffering is arbitrary, pointless and unfair, but knowledge of suffering lived through and overcome can be positive.

As Ivan Illich argues, by medicalizing more and more aspects of our experience we also risk handing over control of more of our lives to professionals. We lose knowledge, autonomy and resilience. Medicalizing ever greater swathes of human experience can also change what it means to be human. Swallowing a pill to annul the pain of loss has the potential to change the meaning of the experience. Through grief we recognize both our own needs and our relations to others. It shows us what we value. We have reasons for our experience, but medicalizing the experience can turn it into aberrant brain chemistry that needs a biochemical fix. We begin to look at ourselves not as experiencing subjects whose feelings have reasons, but as malfunctioning objects in need of fixing.

Autonomy From the Greek for 'self-rule'. Although initially used to refer to independent Greek city-states, it now more generally refers to the ability of individuals to make decisions about their own lives, free from external influence. It is a critical concept in both liberal political theory and medical ethics, where it is associated with the right to make informed choices about medical care.

Labiaplasty A surgical procedure, frequently undertaken for cosmetic purposes, that involves the reshaping of the external female genitalia, specifically the folds of skin surrounding the vulva: the labia minora and labia majora.

Disease mongering The process of widening the boundaries of treatable illness in order to increase the markets for those who sell and provide medical treatments, including drugs and other interventions.

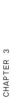

Consider the rise of 'therapeutic' labiaplasty. There is an increase among women, particularly young women, of emotional distress because of perceived abnormalities in the appearance of their labia minora, despite the absence of any organic disorder, and the size of their labia minora falling within the ordinary range. The origins of this distress are multiple, but they include social pressures driven by the proliferation of pornographic imagery in which pubic hair is shaved and women are expected to look pre-pubescent. Although this can be medicalized – anxiety and depression 'treated' with drugs and therapy or surgical reduction – the origins lie with expectations of female appearance. This can create lucrative markets for cosmetic surgery, feed disease mongering and label ever larger numbers of women abnormal.

Should we operate, with all its risks, or consider social change?

A   For cosmetic surgeons, social media can be an incredibly useful platform for the promotion of their services, but it also gives rise to issues of privacy and confidentiality. Here, the Bruna twins display the results of $60,000 of 'free' surgery, paid for by posting images of the results of their treatments on Instagram.

B   The rise of cosmetic surgery such as rhinoplasty for non-therapeutic purposes – improving on normal human appearance – is an increasingly lucrative industry. But should we medicalize dissatisfaction with our looks or try and address social expectation?

C   An estimated $2.4 billion was spent on plastic surgery in China in 2008. Double eyelid surgery – seen here – is the most popular cosmetic procedure in China and arguably gives a more 'Western' appearance. Patients are therefore exposed to risks in order to meet cultural aspirations.

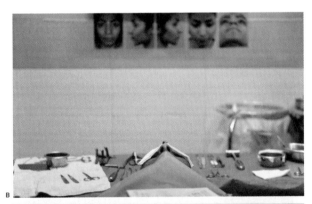
B

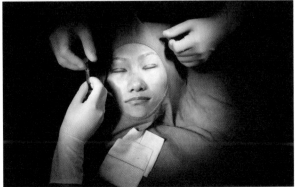
C

Medicalization also increases the costs of health care. Money spent on health cannot be spent on other worthwhile goods, and money spent on trivial or less serious health care is diverted away from those in real need. Every health system in the world struggles with the tension between affordability and equality of access. Privately funded health care may not empty the public purse, but only those who can afford it get the care – and serious illness can bankrupt all but the wealthiest. Publicly funded health care is more equitable, but costs are rising and medicalization is helping drive them.

Other aspects of the natural human lifecycle are also open to medicalization. Is old age, for example, a medical condition? Should it be?

Shakespeare roots old age in nature, a second childhood, 'sans eyes, sans teeth, sans taste, sans everything'. But modern Western culture is increasingly at war with it, and we arm ourselves with medicine. The most natural and, if we live long enough, inevitable life stage is now a permanent medical condition, and a massive marketplace.

In his book *The Medicalization of Society* (2007), US sociologist Peter Conrad gives a fine account of the medicalization of ageing. Although he concentrates on the medicalization of masculinity, his ideas cross gender boundaries. For Conrad, the medicalization of age is driven by a desire to retain the attractive physical and cognitive capacities of youth and middle age: vigour, tone, sexual potency, mental alacrity, a full head of hair. But it is also driven by fear – and distaste – for age.

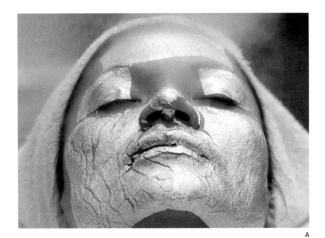

A

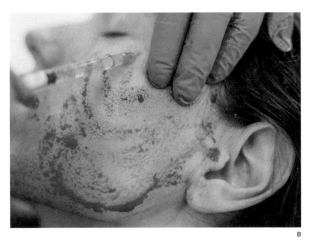

B

A   Old age and the changes in
the human body associated
with it are increasingly seen as
medical phenomena. Here, gold
leaf is applied to the face as an
alleged anti-ageing treatment.
B   The search for eternal youth
is hardly new, but there is
a plethora of novel – and
evidence-free – interventions,
such as the vampire facial.

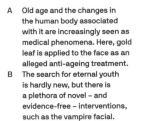

The ravages of old age may never have
been welcome, although the great French
essayist Michel de Montaigne thought they
were a useful instruction in how to die, but
modern Western society is increasingly at
odds with ageing. Ours is an ageist society,
seeing only loss in growing old. To counter
our decline, or to try and take some control
over it, we turn to medical technology. And
if medicine can fix the problem, it seems
to follow that it must have been a medical
problem in the first place. What we once
saw as a natural process – changes in the
hair and skin – has become pathological.
We are not just old; we are diseased.

Unlike some classic early accounts of the medicalization of the female body, which focused on medical imperialism – particularly the expansion of male medical control over the female body – the medicalization of masculinity has several drivers. Men, keen to slow down the effects of ageing, conspire in it.

Medical imperialism The process of extending the power or reach of medical explanation or dominion over increasingly large swathes of human experience that have previously been understood as ordinary or natural features.

Psychogenic Brought about by the mind. Usually refers to physical ailments whose origin lies in emotional or psychological distress or psychiatric disorders.

There is a huge market for potency-enhancing drugs and hair loss treatment. Conscious of this, pharmaceutical companies seek products to meet the need. Viagra (sildenafil citrate) is the fastest selling drug of all time. It started life as a proposed treatment for angina. It didn't work, but research participants noticed an intriguing side effect: erections. The drug company, Pfizer, had stumbled upon a goldmine.

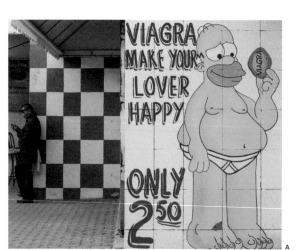

VIAGRA MAKE YOUR LOVER HAPPY ONLY 2⁵⁰

A The attempt to overcome the downsides of male ageing, including declining sexual potency, has opened up new dimensions of medicalization, with male consumers driving demand. Viagra, a drug intended for those with pathological erectile problems, has rapidly become a fully fledged lifestyle drug.
B Drug manufacturers see a lucrative market in giving people what they want, including eternal virility. However, the success of drugs such as Viagra has led to counterfeit brands being sold by unscrupulous pharmacies around the world.

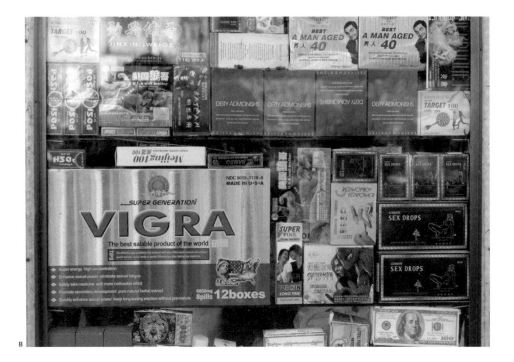

B

The role of the medical profession in this process was muted. In Britain, Viagra was initially a prescription-only medicine. Its early use was restricted to those whose erectile dysfunction was linked to prostate cancer, diabetes or renal failure, although there was pressure from patients to broaden access. It can now be bought over the counter in Britain.

Because the therapeutic, performance-enhancing benefits of Viagra are so desirable, it nicely portrays the way a medical intervention that was initially focused on conditions that most agree are 'serious' or clinical begins to widen.

From those whose dysfunction is organic, it was used for those whose erectile problem, though serious, had no obvious physical cause and was likely to be psychogenic. It was then used for those with occasional, less serious erectile issues. Now, it is a fully fledged lifestyle drug, enhancing the erections of those who do not see themselves as ill or dysfunctional.

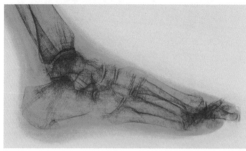

The andropause, or 'male menopause', is associated with a cluster of unwelcome changes experienced by some men in their late 40s and early 50s. They include depression, loss of libido, erectile dysfunction, loss of muscle mass, gynaecomastia (man boobs), mood swings, irritability, loss of energy, insomnia and difficulties in concentrating. In the USA, prescription of testosterone to address these symptoms is widespread, but there is medical uncertainty about whether the andropause exists. In men, there is no sudden middle-aged slump in testosterone. Its age-related decline is gradual: less than 2% a year. Conrad describes how, following the isolation of testosterone in 1935, drug companies were actively in search of a market for it. Conditions that seemed to require intervention more urgently, such as sexual underdevelopment, were too small a market. But there was gold in male mid-life change.

There are similar issues with the medicalization of female ageing.

Declining oestrogen levels were designated a marker of disease – the menopause – for which the treatment was hormone replacement therapy (HRT).

Not only could HRT relieve symptoms of this 'disease', it could also rescue women from the physical changes that come with age, transforming them into a disease for which HRT was the cure. By 1975, HRT was the fifth most commonly prescribed drug in the USA. Conrad also draws stark attention to the downside of medicalization: despite heavy promotion, early HRT was not risk-free. There were links to certain cancers, and by 1979 its use was rapidly declining. Similarly, concerns were raised about its 'safer' replacement, a combination of oestrogen and progestin, again heavily promoted by drug companies. By 2001, 33% of US women over the age of 50 were taking the new HRT. However, a study published in 2002 in the *Journal of the American Medical Association* turned everything upside down. An eight-year clinical trial comparing HRT to placebo was suspended after identifying significant risks of breast cancer, blood clots and heart disease. A later study showed no improvements in quality of life.

HRT remains controversial. Although many women experience significant benefits – and recent research suggests there is no association between HRT and increased mortality – there are still risks. In its early days, despite heavy marketing and redemptive promises, the medicalization of menopause was very nearly catastrophic.

Menopause A natural part of female ageing associated with declining oestrogen levels. In most women, the menopause occurs between 45 and 55 years of age. Many women experience unpleasant side effects, including hot flushes, night sweats, declining libido, low moods and anxiety. Menopause is frequently seen as an area of medicalization.

B

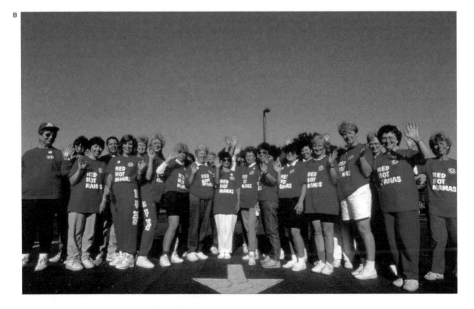

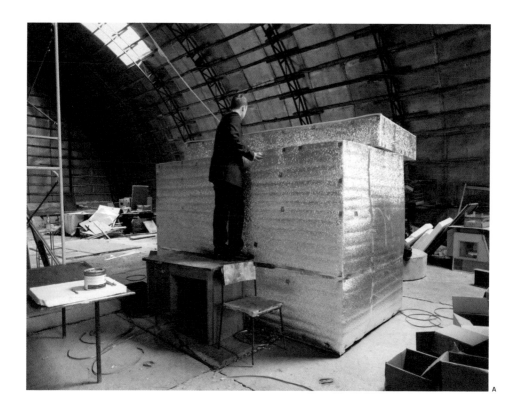

A

Nowhere are the paradoxes of medicalization more intense than at the end of life.

A/B Death is increasingly medicalized and the almost miraculous powers of modern medicine lead some to believe that death can be overcome. In our modern litigious culture, pressure on doctors to ensure that everything possible has been done to preserve life is intense. Seen here are liquid nitrogen-filled human storage units at KrioRus, just outside Moscow. Full bodies and heads are stored in metal vats, in the hope that they might be revived one day and return to life.

There is a moving account in the medical press by a doctor who was himself a doctor's son. As he was growing up and training, his father talked to him about patients who refused to accept the inevitability of death. On the very lip of it, they clamoured for every last intervention, grasped at the frailest straws, clutched at anything to put off the terrible end. He could not understand why they refused to accept the inevitable.

Yet, despite all his protestations, when it was his turn to die, he did the same thing: anything, absolutely anything, to hang on for a few more breaths.

For the foreseeable future, death is still inevitable. As the span of our lives increases, the more likely we are to suffer from multiple illnesses as we approach it. For each of these illnesses, we seek interventions that have side effects. And for these side effects, we seek further interventions. A medical landslide can follow.

There is also the impact of misplaced scientific optimism. If death is a medical phenomenon, the result of disease or injury, then there is always a possibility of a technological fix, if not now then soon, a result of those 'medical advances' that are never out of the media. On this view, death is not a natural and inevitable event, but a medical failure, something that could have been avoided.

Much modern medicine is also risk averse. Western cultures are increasingly litigious. And if death is the ultimate medical risk, it is little wonder that professional pressure to avoid it is intense. This helps explain why so many of us now die in intensive care: if the lawyers come knocking, at least everything possible was tried.

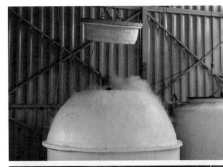
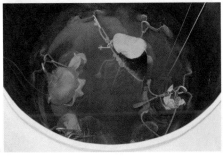

B

But given that death is inevitable, how do we want to go about it? What would a good death look like? Most of us would want it to be as pain- and anguish-free as possible. But how 'medical' do we want it to be? How technological? Do we want to die in an intensive treatment unit or would we rather die at home, in the company of family and friends? If that is not possible, would we prefer to go to a hospice, to die among those practised at the humane arts of palliative care? How much emphasis should we give to prolonging the end of our lives, and how much to the quality of it? These questions point to new aspects of medicalization.

Death is now, overwhelmingly, a medical phenomenon.

Hospice Both a form and philosophy of care usually made available for those with a terminal illness for whom curative, hospital-based interventions are no longer appropriate. It usually involves both symptom management and a careful attention to emotional and spiritual needs at the end of a patient's life.

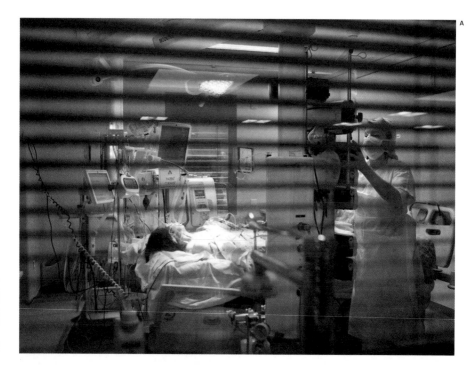

A

A Although the desire to extend life is central to medicine, deciding when to stop active – and burdensome – treatment in an intensive care unit, for example, is critical to ensuring a good death.

B Increasingly, those living in more affluent countries die outside their homes, in hospitals and other caring institutions. Although medical care and support can be excellent, arguably the institutionalization of death has removed it from ordinary experience. Here, pills are sorted into a weekly dispenser for a patient in a German nursing home.

Doctors will likely tell us when and where in the body it started. They will probably tell us when it will come. They will do everything they can to defer it, and to smooth our passage, and then certify to the world that it came. At the beginning of the 19th century, almost all of us died at home. Now more than 80% of Americans die in a medical institution, and as many as 60% in acute hospitals.

Yet death is no more an illness than birth.

It is the most human of events. And what happens to our understanding of ourselves if we consign our deaths to professionals? How can we make sense of it?

Medicalization and its paradoxes lie at the complex heart of the forces driving modern medicine. Some reap unalloyed benefits; others push it in directions that are harmful, both economically and in terms of individual health and well-being. Commercial actors are critical. Drug and medical device companies want to expand their markets.

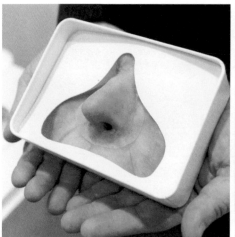
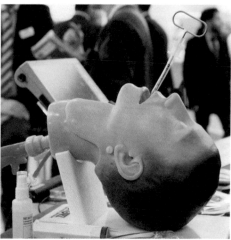

A

In the 1970s, Henry Gadsden, then chief executive of the pharmaceutical giant Merck, told *Fortune* magazine about his frustration that medicines were only sold to the sick. He wanted drugs to be as widely used as Wrigley's chewing gum. His ambition was to sell his drugs to everyone. Not only did Gadsden quadruple Merck's revenue, he transformed the way Westerners think about health and illness. Unleashing the full arsenal of modern marketing techniques, exploiting fears of illness, loneliness, suffering and ageing, demand for medicines, particularly among healthy Americans, went through the roof. There was, in theory, nobody, no matter how apparently healthy, that they could not induce to take medicines.

Allied to this are rising expectations, partly driven by commercial marketing, partly by medicine's extraordinary successes. Illness and suffering are increasingly seen as aberrations or failures, unwarranted interruptions in lives where health, happiness and a congenial old age are birth rights.

Even if you are not obviously unwell, why settle for the hand that nature allotted you? If a good life is contingent upon excellences of body and mind, and medical technology can improve on them, why should we not exploit them?

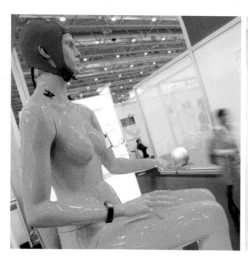
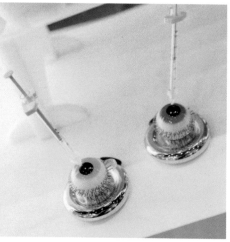

Why not demand the enhancements necessary for us to thrive in the jungle of modern capitalism, with its competitiveness, materialism and hyper-individualism?

Hyper-individualism
Whereas individualism prioritizes both the moral importance of the individual and the obligation to maximize individual flourishing, hyper-individualism recognizes no restraints on individual self-promotion arising from the common or public good.

Combine these forces with commercial pay-for-service health delivery and the grounds have been laid for a massive expansion in medical interventions – much of it unnecessary, some of it, inevitably, harmful.

If there is one area where the impact of medicalization, and the enormous increase in medical interventions that attend it, is starkest, it is in relation to cost. As we will see in Chapter 4, modern medicine, on its current trajectory and driven by its current assumptions, is unaffordable.

Something has to change.

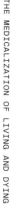

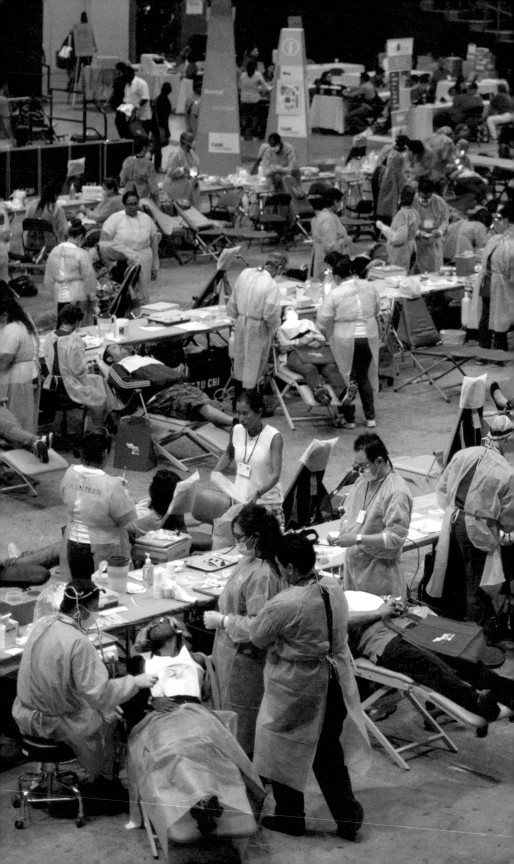

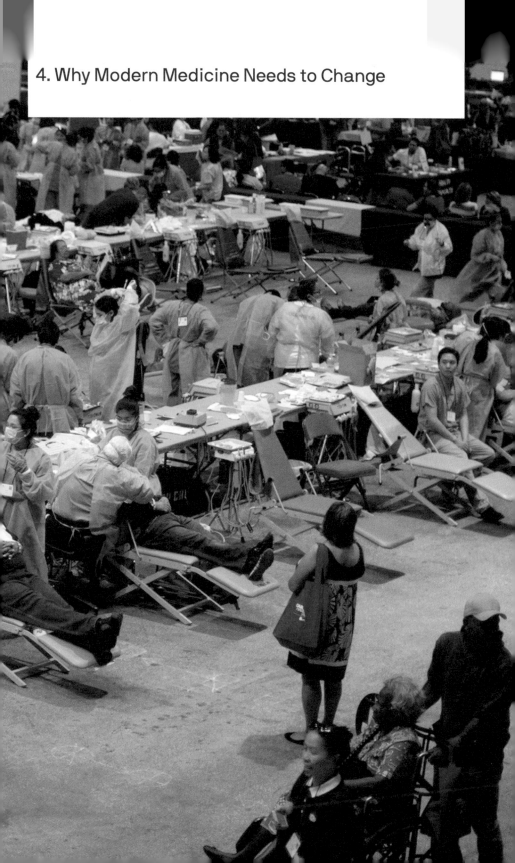

4. Why Modern Medicine Needs to Change

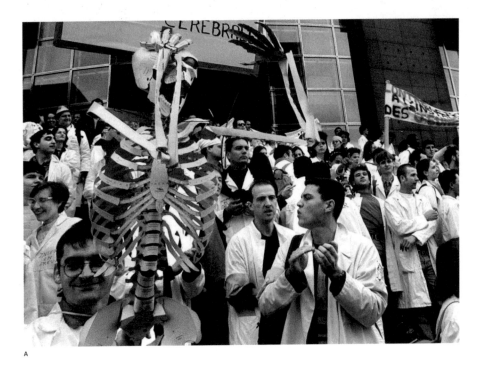

A

In early 2018, the US drug company Spark Therapeutics announced the introduction of a new genetic therapy for treating certain types of inherited retinal degeneration that lead to blindness. It involves a one-off injection into each eye using a virus to insert a replacement gene. The therapy, called Luxturna, costs $425,000 per injection – a total of $850,000 for the full treatment.

A   Ageing populations, high-tech medicine and rising expectations drive up the costs of medicine, making medicine a major political issue. Here, French doctors protest government spending plans, which challenge their freedom to consult and prescribe as they wish.

B   Although pharmaceutical companies are major global players and profits can be enormous, research and development into new drugs is expensive and risky. Here, workers from Teva Pharmaceutical Industries block roads to protest staff layoffs in Israel in 2017.

The biggest practical problem confronting medicine is cost. How can we pay for it?

Every country in the world, irrespective of its wealth, size or chosen model of payment and delivery, wrestles with this question.

Comparing the way countries deal with health costs is not straight-forward. Although most have their own idiosyncrasies, they draw on and frequently combine several basic models of payment and delivery.

At one end of the spectrum – India and the USA are good examples – there is overwhelming reliance on private payment, whether directly or via private or employer-based insurance programmes. This is combined with private delivery of health services via commercial health providers. Although this frees up public funds, there are serious drawbacks in relation to fairness, equality and cost.

Most mainland European countries – and many others – favour some form of social health insurance (SHI). Those at work, and usually their employers, pay into a mutual fund that provides them and their dependants with a package of health benefits. Treatment is either free at the point of care or involves a degree of co-payment. Governments frequently make contributions, improving the range of benefits and ensuring financial stability. Many SHI schemes are extended to cover those who are unable to pay into them. They usually involve some form of progressive transfer of funds from rich to poor, and risks are often pooled: the sick seldom pay more than the well, and risks are spread across the lifecycle. Health services can be delivered by commercial, not-for-profit or state-run organizations, or some combination.

Social health insurance (SHI)
A mechanism for funding health provision. Typically, employees and their employers pay into an insurance fund that provides them, and their dependants, with a defined package of health services. Contributions are usually compulsory, and many governments subsidize them to ensure financial stability.

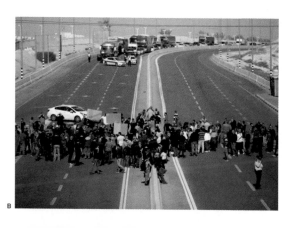

B

Elective surgery From the Latin *eligere* (to choose). Refers to surgery that is planned in advance as it is not immediately necessary in order to save the patient's life or to prevent serious deterioration.

Gross domestic product (GDP) An economic term referring to the total value of all the goods and services produced by an individual country, usually measured in a single year.

Economic ultra-liberalism A form of extreme, often ideological commitment to free market and laissez-faire economic policies. According to this view, the maximum possible number of economic decisions should be made by private individuals and households, with a minimum of state involvement.

At the other end lie national health systems. Revenue is usually raised by direct compulsory taxation, and health coverage is universal and free at the point of delivery. Most services are provided directly by the state. Although Britain is often cited as an example of this system, commercial suppliers and competitive practices are increasingly features of its National Health Service (NHS).

Whichever model a country favours, the forces outlined in this book are whipping up a perfect economic and political storm in the provision of health services. In England, the NHS is in a state of almost permanent political siege. During the winter of 2017–18, all elective surgery was closed due to excessive demand arising from entirely predictable winter pressures. Waiting lists are growing, health staff are under unprecedented strain and crisis has become permanent, with doctors complaining of 'Third World conditions'. Meanwhile, dissatisfaction among patients and medical staff grows. It feels as if something must give.

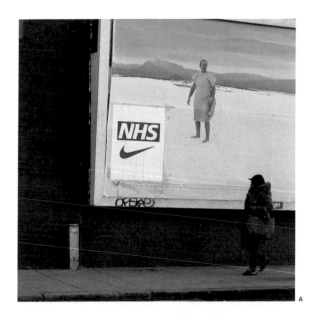

A   Attempts to reduce costs in the NHS have led to experimentation with commercial models, which has stoked political disagreement. This politically provocative NHS/Nike poster by Jonny Banger (Sports Banger) was created as part of the junior doctors protest campaign. Here, it is pasted on top of a Macmillan poster, reading 'Cancer can be the loneliest place'.

B   Although health care in the USA can be excellent, it is characterized by high costs, poor and socially unjust coverage, and low patient satisfaction. Attempts to widen access, such as Obamacare – advertised here at an insurance store in California – have been politically divisive.

A

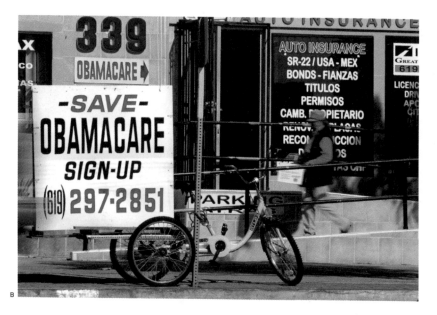

In the USA, where the market is the norm, the situation is dire. Health care costs are stratospheric, pushing towards one-fifth of US gross domestic product (GDP). Health is a divisive political football, with individualism, economic ultra-liberalism and deep suspicion of the state making top-down political change difficult. But leaving payment of health care insurance to private individuals or their employers, and delivery to commercial organizations, means large numbers of people are partially or totally uninsured. Costs are out of control. If you are wealthy, it is possible to get exceptional medical care in the USA, but the system is unjust, expensive and inefficient. Poverty, for example, rules out access to good health care.

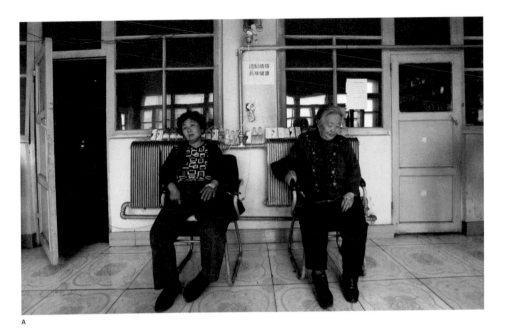

A

A   Despite extraordinary economic growth, China has serious challenges in ensuring access to good health care outside the major cities. This rural medical clinic cares for around 600,000 patients, who live in the areas surrounding the city of Shuangcheng.

B   Access to primary health care services in remote areas of India remains limited. Here, doctors perform surgery in an operating theatre on the Lifeline Express, a hospital built inside a seven-coach train, at a railway station in Jalore.

Then there are the challenges facing the two most populous countries in the world: China and India.

Nearly 1.4 billion people live in China. In 2014, it spent 5.5% of GDP on health. Explosive economic growth has lifted many out of poverty and overall health outcomes have improved. Wealthy city-dwellers have access to high-tech health services, but many rural poor have no access to even basic health care provision. Despite nearly half the population living in rural areas, government investment is heavily skewed towards cities: around 80% of medical services are concentrated in metropolitan areas. There is a chronic lack of public health infrastructure in rural areas, with as much as 80% of rural poor lacking access to sanitation and 20% lacking safe drinking water. There is also significant variation in the skills and education of health professionals, pay-for-service health provision drives expensive over-treatment, and out-of-pocket payments for health can be financially devastating. In addition, rapid economic growth has led to significant environmental degradation, stacking up health problems for the future.

India, with a population in the region of 1.3 billion, spends even less than China on health: 4.7% of GDP. Whereas China's public spend on health is 3.1% of GDP, India's is only 1.4%. Despite India's constitution guaranteeing universal health care to all, in 2014, 62.4% of health spending was out-of-pocket because publicly provided health care is shunned due to poor quality and lack of availability. Private health provision dominates.

According to an article in *The Times of India* (2015), every year 63 million people are forced below the poverty line due to catastrophic expenditure on health care.

Like China, India's health services are focused on urban areas. A crucial health challenge is rural-to-urban migration, which can overwhelm health care infrastructure in destination cities. Despite the strong reliance on private health provision, three-quarters of the population have no insurance coverage.

Environmental degradation
The process by which the natural environment is depleted, damaged or degraded such that biodiversity is reduced, habitat is damaged, and natural resources such as air and water are polluted. It is usually said to be the result of human activity.

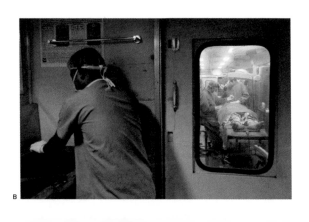

B

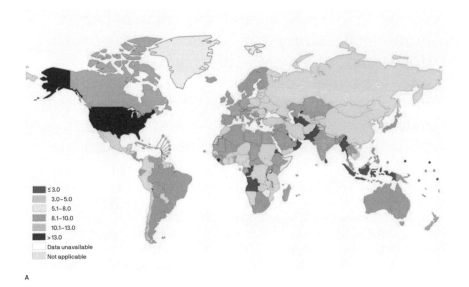

Before going further, we need to look at what economists call opportunity costs. Every pound spent on health is a pound that cannot be spent on other good things. Health is vitally important; it is a foundational human good. But so too are education, the environment in which we live, justice and freedom, and national security. Understandably, we rank our health highly when it is at risk, but when we are feeling better we remember the importance of the things we live for.

Despite what the media might have us think, there is more to life than good health. It is a means, not an end.

A Globally, there are huge variations in health care spending. Although wealthier countries spend more, this is not always equated with better overall health outcomes. This map shows total expenditure on health as a percentage of GDP in 2011.

B Different countries adopt different economic models of health care provision. The USA spends the highest proportion of GDP on health, but much of this is private payment. This map shows general government expenditure on health as a percentage of total expenditure in 2011.

Opportunity costs A term in economic theory that refers to the cost of the benefit that is foregone as a result of making a choice between alternatives.

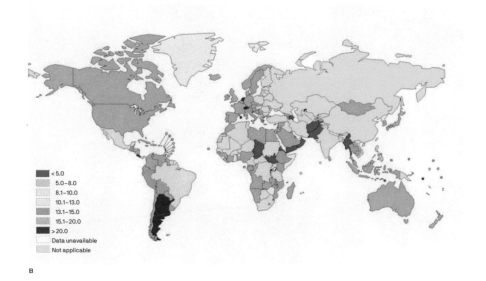

- < 5.0
- 5.0–8.0
- 8.1–10.0
- 10.1–13.0
- 13.1–15.0
- 15.1–20.0
- > 20.0
- Data unavailable
- Not applicable

B

So how much do we spend on health? According to the World Health Organization (WHO), in 2015 the world spent 7.3 trillion US dollars, almost 10% of GDP. (GDP spend on education is closer to 5%). The share of GDP spend on health is biggest in high-income countries, with an average of around 12%, and lowest in middle-income countries, at 6%. In low-income countries, where health needs are usually the highest, it sits at around 7%. Among the 35 member countries of the Organisation for Economic Co-operation and Development (OECD), the average is around 9%.

The USA spends by far the largest percentage of GDP on health, a colossal 17.9% in 2016. (In 2014, the USA spent 6.2% of GDP on education). Of the G7 group of leading economies (Canada, France, Germany, Italy, Japan, Britain and the USA), Britain is ranked sixth. British spending on health care in 2014 was £179 billion, or 9.9% of GDP. Italy's was the lowest at 9.1% in 2014. France and Germany spent more than Britain, around 11% of GDP.

Although among the OECD countries there is some correlation between health care expenditure and life expectancy, it is not uniform.

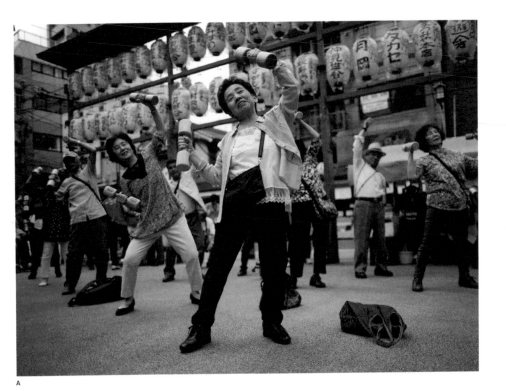

A

In 2016, the USA spent $10,348 (about £7,600) per person on health care; Britain spent $4,192 (about £3,090). Within the G7, in 2014, Japan had the highest life expectancy despite spending only the fifth most per person, while Italy spent the least and had the second highest life expectancy. Average life expectancy at birth in the USA was 78.8 years, but as we have seen, life expectancy has fallen in the USA largely because of the opioid epidemic. In Britain, life expectancy at birth in the same year was 81.4. (Interestingly, for reasons not yet fully understood, life expectancy in Britain is no longer increasing. Some associate this with the cuts in social services linked to 'austerity', but no clear causal link has been established.)

It is not surprising to find no firm correlation between health spend and life expectancy.

Most health spend is remedial, addressing illness after it has arisen. Once the major infectious diseases have been tackled, lifestyle factors – diet, exercise, cigarette and alcohol consumption – and underlying determinants, such as socio-economic gradient and educational attainment, have a bigger impact on longevity. As does gender: in Japan, women live on average six years longer than men. Although rates are reducing, ischaemic heart disease is still the most common cause of death in the OECD countries. Smoking rates are declining, as is the incidence of cancer, but obesity and heavy drinking remain serious public health problems.

Ischaemic heart disease
Also known as coronary heart disease. Refers to the blocking of the bloody supply to the heart following the build-up of fatty deposits in the coronary arteries, a process known as atherosclerosis. It is a major source of global morbidity.

A   Among the key global health challenges is how to tackle the health problems associated with modern lifestyles, including obesity and cardiovascular disease. Here, elderly people exercise in Tokyo.

B   Tackling loneliness among the elderly is a major challenge in parts of Japan; loneliness can itself lead to, or compound, health problems. Events such as the Bon dance in Tokiwadaira provide opportunities to socialize.

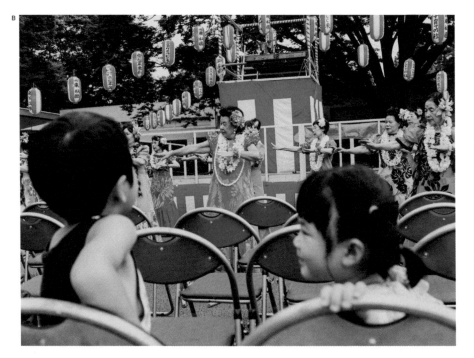

So where does the spend in health go? As a percentage, in all or almost all countries, spending is overwhelmingly directed on after-the-event curative and rehabilitative health services, much of it expensive and with increasing reliance on high-tech interventions. Hospitals, doctor appointments and emergency intervention take the lion's share. As we have seen, commercial organizations, seeking rapid and early penetration for their innovations, are a significant driver of cost. In the USA, somewhere in the region of 50% of the annual increase in US health costs is due to new technology.

But there are other drivers. Some of the pressure for innovation comes from the influence of 'baby boomers', the generation born in the West after the war that came of age in the 1960s. Compared to earlier generations, baby boomers were wealthy, fit, active, opinionated, politically literate and with a keen sense of entitlement. If medicine is the last – beleaguered – enclave of the enlightenment, the baby boomers are its foot soldiers. They were the first generation to enjoy as standard many of the great medical innovations described in this book: antibiotics, safe surgical procedures, the contraceptive pill. And as they move into their 60s, 70s and 80s, so their optimism – and entitlement – has stayed with them. They make it demonstrably clear that they have a right to whatever health care they require; their lives are as valuable as anybody else's. And if their rights are curtailed, they will make their frustration felt at the ballot box. No wonder this is a nettle politicians find almost impossible to grasp.

As the baby boomer generation moves into old age, its members seek to retain, for as long as possible, their health and mobility. These images of baby boomers enjoying various cruises are from a series titled *Love Boat Rejects* by Ian Hughes. Most health care costs are concentrated in the last years of life, often involving multiple health problems and their associated medications. How to afford the health care needs of an ageing population is a challenge faced by all economically developed countries.

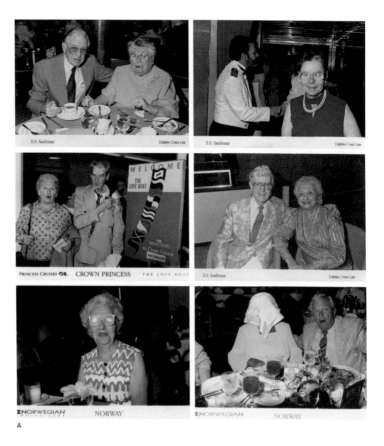

A

There are also rising concerns about the expensive, and all too often counterproductive, over-medicalization of old age. The British doctor and author James Le Fanu has published numerous compelling stories from his readers about the impact of polypharmacy. He speaks of elderly victims of a 'prescribing cascade', in which every prescribed drug requires another one to respond to its side effects, often interacting with frightening results. According to Le Fanu, adverse drug reactions have been reported in 44% of hospital inpatients and make up 10% of emergency hospital admissions.

Age is also where the economic challenge is sharpest.

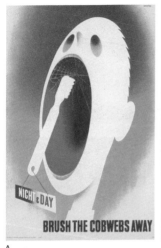
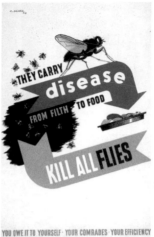
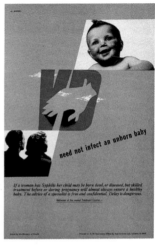

A

In 2016, more than two-fifths of NHS spending in Britain was devoted to people over the age of 65. An 85-year-old man will cost the NHS about seven times as much as a man in his late 30s: an average of £7,000 a year. And this age weighting will only increase. According to the British Office of National Statistics, on current trends, by 2039 almost a quarter of the population will be over the age of 65, with one in 12 over 80. In the USA, research indicates that in 2013, more than 36% of lifetime health care costs were spent on those over 65, largely on ischaemic heart disease, diabetes and hypertension. (Compare this to government public health spending for the same year: an estimated $77.9 billion, or about 2.8% of total health spending.)

This loading of health care costs towards the end of life, combined with our obsession with the dazzle of medical technology, leads us, tragically, to neglect the origins of health and well being. In many Western states, liberal individualism and a suspicion of the state make it politically difficult to look at collective change in relation to the origins of good health. In Britain, approximately 5% of the total health budget is spent on public health services, such as health promotion and the management of environmental hazards. And that figure is declining. In the USA, in 2014, it was 2.65%, and again that percentage was expected to fall. Approximately half of OECD countries have reduced public health spending in the past five years.

This leaves us on the horns of a dilemma, one laid out by the US philosopher Daniel Callahan in his book *Taming the Beloved Beast* (2009). If each of us has a reasonable claim to health services in accordance with our needs, then health care costs will bunch towards the end of life. Although there was optimistic talk about 'compression of morbidity' – a long and comparatively healthy life with a small tail of illness right at the end – this looks less plausible. Increasing co-morbidities and polypharmacy are more likely. Given cost pressures, more of our resources will be spent providing care in the final years, with an intense burst in the last weeks and months. But should so much of our collective economic good be concentrated here, particularly if the war against ageing, ill health and death is unwinnable? How should we adjudicate between the needs of our older population and the needs of children and adults starting out in their lives, or in their middle years? It may sound brutal, but is the sole purpose of our common good the prolongation of the final years of our lives?

Liberal individualism
A political position predicated on the belief that individuals should be maximally free to pursue their own self-realization with minimal interference from the state. The interests of the individual are regarded as prior to the interests of the group or state.

A   Although prevention is better than cure – as these public health posters by Abram Games testify – the elimination of many early health threats has led to a significant increase in age-related morbidity.

B   These Chinese public health posters are from the 1950s. Today, the rise of political individualism and its associated suspicion of state intervention make government public health interventions contentious.

B

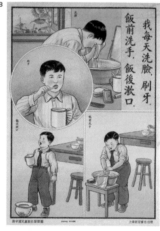

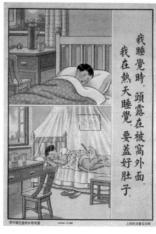

Jen Sinconis and her husband were well-to-do, middle-class Americans. Pregnant with twins, she went into labour at 24 weeks. Her twin boys weighed just over a pound each and spent the next six months in the neonatal intensive care unit (Nicu). The boys suffered many of the health problems associated with extreme premature birth, including cerebral palsy, brain haemorrhages, jaundice and heart defects. Writing in the British *Guardian* newspaper, she recounts the family's descent into debt as a bed in the Nicu costs $10,000 dollars a night. Many of the treatments the boys required were not covered by their insurance policy, and after 18 months they had hit the $2 million cap on their policy. $450,000 in debt, the couple sold everything they owned and filed for bankruptcy.

There is a great deal to learn about modern health care and its economic challenges by looking at the USA.

On the plus side, those who have sufficient money or effective health insurance can probably get some of the best health care in the world in the USA. Treatment for specialist conditions in leading US hospitals can be exceptional. If you have the right coverage, or can afford to pay, waiting times in the USA are short and choice is vast. There is huge investment in medical research and state-of-the-art medical technology.

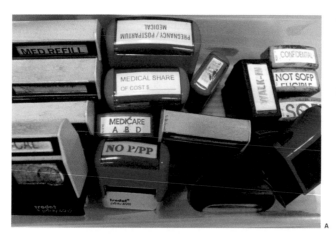

A The USA spends the largest percentage of GDP on health globally for less than universal coverage. Here, stamps are used to classify patient documents.
B One aspect of US culture is an unhealthy relationship with readily available fast food and junk food, such as this donut diner. Nearly 30% of Americans are obese, which can lead to a cascade of serious health problems.

A

Infant mortality The ratio of the number of deaths in the first year of life to the number of live births in the same population during the same time. It is usually expressed as a ratio per 1,000 live births in a year.

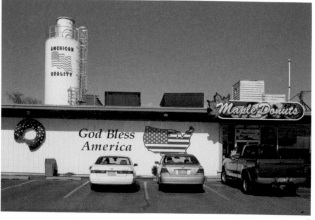

B

But there is a downside. Despite spending nearly twice the OECD average on health, the USA has low overall life expectancy. Taken at a population level, the US health care system is appallingly inefficient. By almost all standards of comparison, US health care is worse than other high-income countries. Infant mortality, a vital indicator, is around 7 deaths per 1,000 live births; in Finland it is 2. The USA spends about eight times as much per capita on health as Qatar, for a single year's gain in life expectancy.

The USA is also among the most unequal of modern wealthy countries. There is increasing evidence to suggest that social inequalities contribute to poorer health outcomes. The work of Sir Michael Marmot and others has established a clear social gradient in health: the higher up the social ladder, the better your overall health outcomes are likely to be. In *The Spirit Level* (2009), Kate Pickett and Richard Wilkinson argue that inequality is itself a strong driver of ill health.

Perversely, by some metrics, the USA is among the unhealthiest nations in the world. It tops the global obesity statistics. In 2015, over a third of Americans aged 15 or over were obese, as were 31% of children. And obesity is strongly correlated with heart disease, diabetes, a range of cancers and musculo-skeletal problems. The economic cost of obesity in the USA is somewhere between $147 billion and $210 billion a year.

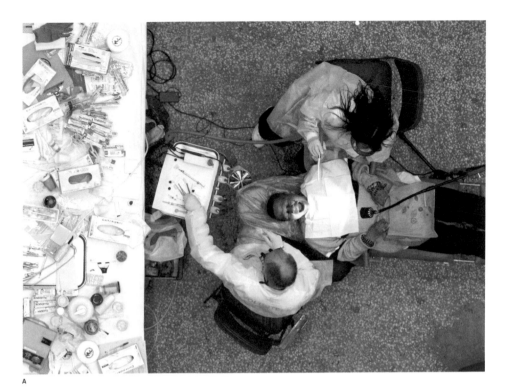

A

A/B Patients receive dental treatment at the Remote Area Medical clinic in Los Angeles in 2010. This non-profit organization provides free medical, dental and vision care via mobile clinics. Arguably, the biggest shortcoming of the US health system is its lack of universal coverage. A single serious episode of ill health can lead to bankruptcy. Even among insured patients, sustained ill health can exhaust the insurance policy, leading to personal liability for costs and serious economic hardship, including homelessness.

But its greatest problem is coverage. At the beginning of 2018, Bloomberg ran a story about three fairly typical working families in the USA. By no means poor, all three families – the Buchanans from Marion, North Carolina, the Owens from Harahan, New Orleans, and the Bobbies from Phoenix, Arizona – decided they could no longer afford their monthly $1,800 plus insurance coverage. The three families are now gambling with their futures. A single serious episode of illness, let alone having to deal with premature twins like Jen Sinconis, could bankrupt them – and their plight is repeated across the USA.

According to the US Centers for Disease Control and Prevention (CDC), in 2016 just over 28 million people under the age of 65, or 10.4% of the population, had no health insurance. Some 5.1% of children under the age of 18 were uninsured, as were 12.4% of those aged 18 to 64.

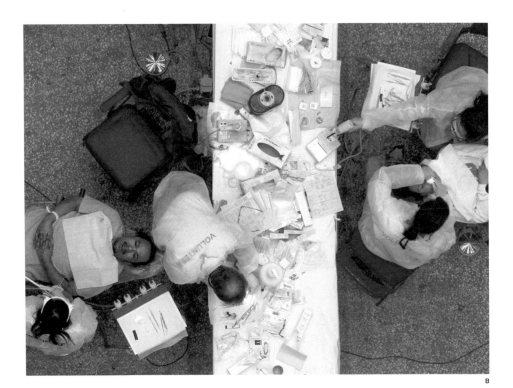

There is also a strong ethnic dimension. In 2014, more than a third of Hispanic adults between the ages of 18 and 64 were uninsured, 17.6% of non-Hispanic black compared to 14.5% of non-Hispanic white and 12.1% of non-Hispanic Asian. Unsurprisingly, this is reflected in health outcomes. According to the WHO, infants born to African American women are two to three times more likely to die than those born to women of other races or ethnicities. US men of all ages and ethnicities are four times more likely to die by suicide than women. African American men are most likely to develop cancer – a rate of 598.5 per 100,000.

For those who are uninsured, like the Owens, Bobbies and Buchanans, and who cannot otherwise afford access to good health care, a single episode of ill health in the family can be devastating. For those on low wages, the choice is stark: to risk bankruptcy through trying to pay for health care or risk unemployment through ill health. The negative feedback loop between poverty and health routinely devastates lives across generations.

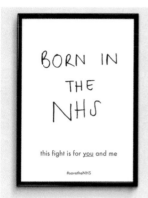
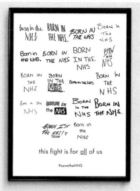
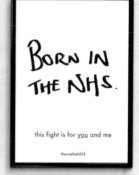

A

To add final insult to injury, Americans do not like their health care system. They routinely poll among the most dissatisfied of wealthy nations. Americans are unlikely to have primary care doctors. Care is badly coordinated, inconvenient and risky, and there are high rates of iatrogenic harms in US health care. Incentives are perverse throughout the system: doctors are not rewarded for quality, and patients regularly complain that their doctors do not listen to them.

By contrast, the NHS in Britain has been described, by the Conservative politician Nigel Lawson, as the closest the English come to a religion.

The overwhelming strength of the NHS is that nobody must pay out of their pocket, or via insurance, if they get sick. Nor does it matter what they sicken from; unlike a lot of private health insurance, there are no exclusions. The NHS is both universal – everyone ordinarily resident in Britain is entitled to it – and, with tiny exceptions such as prescription charges, free at the point of need.

In the summer of 2017, in the year of his 75th birthday, Stephen Hawking (1942–2018), the British physicist, cosmologist and author who suffered from a rare form of early onset motor neurone disease, wrote a powerful defence of the NHS. Without it, he would not have survived. The care that he received enabled him, he wrote, to 'live my life as I want and to contribute major advances to our understanding of the universe'.

Primary care Usually the first point of contact between a patient and health services, provided by general practitioners, pharmacists, dentists and opticians. It is usually contrasted with secondary care, which is provided by a specialist upon referral from primary care.

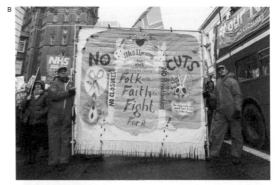
B

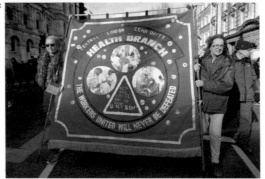
C

A   The NHS is a much-loved institution. It provides near universal coverage, free at the point of care, and is held up as a shining example of social justice. These Born in the NHS posters were created by Carys Norfor in 2016 for her Save the NHS project.

B/C   Rising health costs and efficiency seeking have led successive British governments to experiment with commercial models in the NHS. Concerns about creeping privatization have led to political controversy and organized protest.

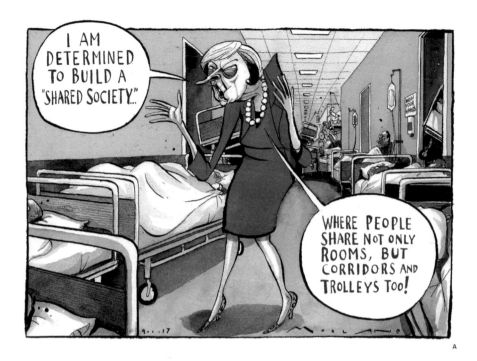

A

Distributive justice
Refers to the justice or fairness of any particular allocation of social goods within a specified group. Theories of distributive justice will seek to specify what allocation or allocations of goods is just or fair.

Moral hazard An economic term referring to circumstances in which an individual or party is more likely to accept risk where they know that they are protected against it because other parties will carry the cost. Moral hazard was said to be in play during the 2007–08 financial crisis because banks were willing to accept high risks, secure in the belief that governments would not let them fail.

The NHS is an exercise in distributive justice. As in Hawking's case, a lot of ill health is a matter of bad luck – genetic or circumstantial. And because, statistically, the lower down the social ladder you are, the greater the risk of ill health, the NHS tends to distribute goods towards the less well off. Sickness in Britain does not spell financial disaster. In comparison to the USA, it is both fair *and* efficient. (Something like half of all personal bankruptcies in the USA are triggered by health care debts.) In 2015, Britain spent just shy of 10% of GDP on health to provide universal, largely state-of-the-art health coverage to its citizens. In the USA, it was 18% for far less universal reach.

But for all its strengths – it is lauded throughout most of the world – the NHS has serious problems, and they go to the heart of what ails modern medicine.

There are unending political battles in Britain, particularly in England, about how the NHS should be funded. Because health needs and costs rise inexorably but available services remain largely fixed, rationing is inevitable. Because neither 'universal' nor 'free at the point of delivery' can be sacrificed, rationing turns into waiting lists. Waiting times grow and frustration builds. The search for efficiency savings intensifies and systems come under pressure. To this is added the problems native to single public providers like the NHS: choice for service users is often poor. There is little inherent pressure to innovate or manage costs. Because care is free, it can be undervalued and squandered. There is also moral hazard: if we do not pay for our own care, there is less incentive for us to manage our conditions.

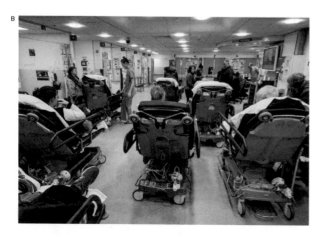

B

A   Political cartoonist Morten Mørland satirizes British Prime Minister Theresa May and her attempts to deal with the financial crisis faced by the NHS.

B   Severe financial pressures in the NHS mean that there is seldom excess capacity. Predictable increases in demand, such as respiratory infections in winter, can rapidly overwhelm available health services, leading, as here, to long waits in hospital corridors.

If we look outside the global West, a different set of economic problems looms.

Consider schistosomiasis, also known as snail fever. It is a disease caused by parasitic worms that live in freshwater in tropical and subtropical zones. Entering the body by burrowing through the skin, the worms move through the blood and lay eggs in the bowels and bladder. Although short-term symptoms include fever, muscle pain and diarrhoea, long term it can lead to death through liver disease and bladder cancer. Usually schistosomiasis can be treated easily and cheaply with the drug praziquantel: a treatment regime costs somewhere between 20 and 30 US cents. Yet there are currently more than 200 million people, mostly in Africa, suffering from the disease.

Nowhere is the failure of the global health system, and the medical-industrial complex that supports it, plainer than in the global distribution of health and illness.

Although the causes are complex, the statistics make painful reading. Consider some recent figures from the WHO. The average global life expectancy of those born in 2015 is 71.4 years. In Sierra Leone it is 51; in Malawi it is 47; in Japan it is 83. In Chad, one in five children dies before their fifth birthday.

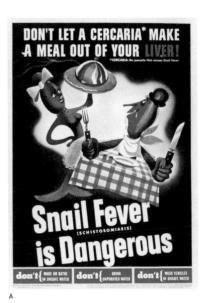

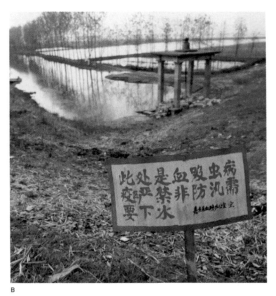

A

B

A/B The burden of ill health arising from preventable water-borne parasitic infections such as snail fever – as seen in this public health poster and Chinese warning – reveal stark inequalities in global health outcomes. These inequalities are an example of market failure. Despite the significant health needs, the lack of purchasing power in the South makes drug research and development economically unattractive.

In Finland, this figure is 2.3 out of every 1,000. In Afghanistan, Somalia and Chad, one woman in 100 dies in childbirth. In 2011, there were no maternal deaths recorded in Finland.

These are the cold outcome statistics, but there are other factors. The WHO estimates that a billion people in the world lack sufficient food – a key determinant of health. Similarly, in the absence of a publicly funded health system, many of the poorest people in the world have to pay for health care out of pocket. Somewhere in the region of 100 million people a year are forced below the poverty line paying for health care. Poverty and ill health are also mutually reinforcing. Poverty is a risk factor for ill health, and ill health is a driver of poverty. And the places with the highest health needs have the lowest concentrations of qualified health professionals. Myanmar and Niger have four doctors for every 100,000 people. Switzerland has 40.

Global health inequities are also a stark reminder of market failure. The poorest people in the world cannot get the care they need, not only because they cannot afford it but also because they make up too small a market to drive innovation.

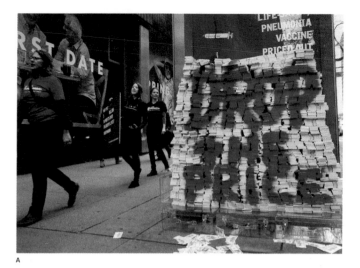

A   The cost of eradication of many of the world's most devastating neglected tropical diseases can be as little as 50 US cents per dose. Here, Doctors Without Borders dumps $17 million in fake money outside Pfizer's HQ to protest high vaccine prices.

B   Tragically, the profitability of medicines and the lack of stringent global oversight for manufacture and distribution of pharmaceuticals lead to counterfeiting of medicines, with potentially devastating consequences for individual and public health. Here, counterfeit drugs are being destroyed.

A

Take neglected tropical diseases (NTDs) such as schistosomiasis. Although largely eradicated in more developed countries, NTDs affect more than a billion people each year, according to estimates by the WHO. Associated with severe illness and disability, the NTDs lock the poorest in the world into a cycle of illness and poverty. The cost to the lowest-income countries runs to billions of dollars, and yet the cost of mass-eradication campaigns for each NTD is about 50 US cents per person per year.

The reasons for neglect are multiple. The infrequency of NTDs in the West enables them to be ignored by the countries with the greatest power to change. Global focus on HIV/AIDS, tuberculosis and malaria – the biggest killers – pushes them down the public health agenda. But the lack of a market means there is no incentive for the big pharmaceutical companies to unleash their huge research and development (R&D) resources. Of the 1,400 drugs registered between 1975 and 1999, less than 1% were for tropical diseases. According to the Drugs for Neglected Diseases Initiative, only 4% of new therapeutic products approved between 2000 and 2011 were for neglected diseases, even though they account for 11% of global diseases. It has been estimated that big pharma invests 90% of its research budget on 10% of diseases. Much commercial pharmaceutical R&D is also focused on 'me-too' drugs: the search for active ingredients similar to existing compounds but with a modified effect. By comparison, R&D for untreated illnesses is regarded as expensive and commercially risky.

The economic problems besetting medicine, though complex and profound, are as much an effect as a cause. Behind them lie deep social attitudes, some of them fostered by medicine, that drive costs inexorably upwards. Put simply, the belief that illness can be overcome, ageing sidestepped and death defeated is false and needs to be set aside. In its place we need to find consensus that, though essential, health is one good among others and cannot, without terrible detriment, be maintained indefinitely.

The forces unleashed by our expectations will, if we are not careful, consume us.

Neglected tropical diseases (NTDs) A complex range of largely parasitical and bacterial diseases concentrated in the 150 or so low-income countries of Asia, Africa and South America. They include Chagas disease, hookworm, human African trypanosomiasis, leishmaniasis and leprosy.

Drugs for Neglected Diseases Initiative A collaborative, not-for-profit research and development organization developing new treatments for neglected diseases globally. It seeks to put patient needs before profit and hence overcome market failure.

B

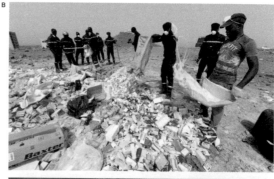

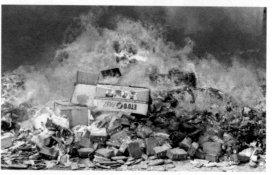

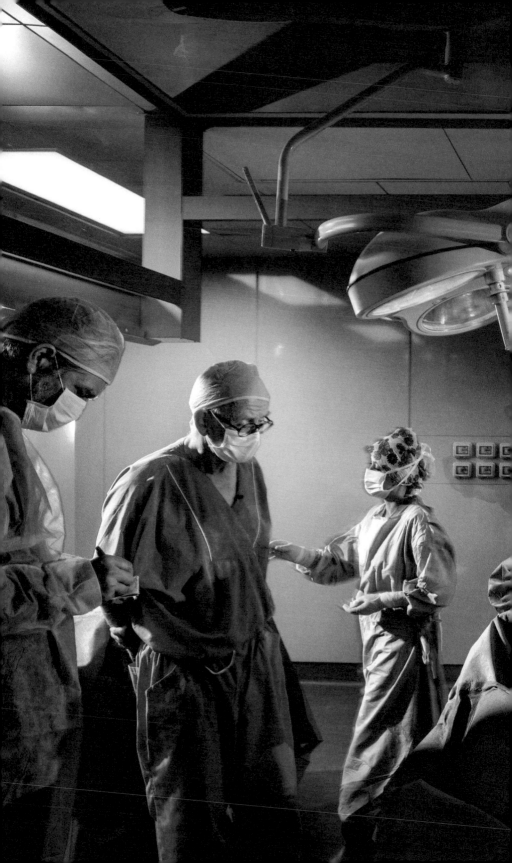

Conclusion

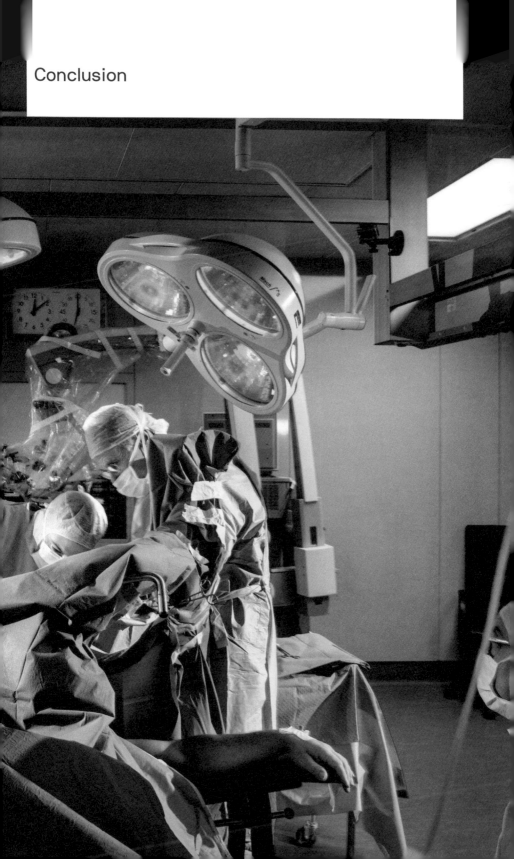

Modern medicine does the most remarkable things.

For those fortunate enough to be able to take it for granted, it is impossible to consider life without it. For thousands of years, the therapeutic cupboard was bare. Now we have anaesthesia, anti-depressants and powerful painkillers. Surgery was once little more than hopeful butchery; now hip replacements are routine and appendicitis, mostly, an inconvenience. There are surgical wonders: heart and lung transplants, brain surgery, the use of robotics. Modern science is unleashing technological marvels: genetic therapies are coming on stream; regenerative medicine is flourishing; lab-grown bladders and tracheas are already helping save lives. There are undersung improvements in day to day care: childbirth has been almost stripped of risk; hospices have transformed end of life care for many.

But for all its wonders, there is a gathering sense that medicine is heading in the wrong direction.

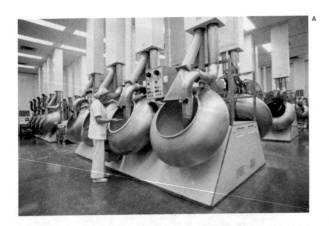

A

A   Despite our increasing reliance on drugs, which are seen being manufactured here, the origins of ill health are often associated with lifestyle.

B   These instructional anatomical dummies are used at a training centre for senior citizen care in Germany. An increasingly ageing population presents great challenges for the economic sustainability of medicine.

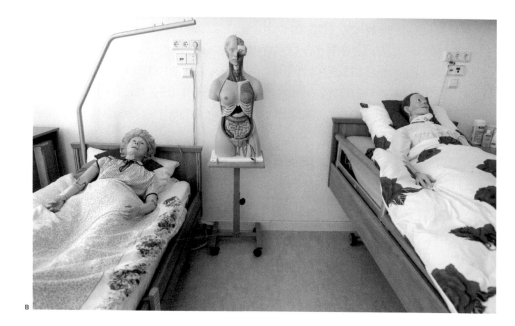

B

Some of this is linked to the unintended consequences of success. Increased life expectancy has not eradicated the need for medicine; it has shifted it elsewhere. Age-related disorders, many of them not curable in the ordinary sense, are proliferating. And much of what we suffer from is not at the cutting edge of high-tech medicine. Not curable in the ordinary sense, a great deal of what ails us requires advice and care as much as advanced medical technology.

After millennia of medical impotence, the first half of the 20th century saw a medical bonanza. Researchers developed an extraordinarily effective arsenal of drugs. Surgical and diagnostic techniques were transformed. Building on the public health gains of the previous century, life expectancy in the West rocketed. But despite the dazzling technology, overall health gains are becoming increasingly marginal – and the costs often formidable.

To this is added the medicalization of human experience, the turn to medicine for quick fixes for a range of human ills. ADHD, alcoholism, infertility, obesity, even death itself are all falling under medicine's inexorably expanding aegis.

Commercial forces are also at work. Medicine is an enormous, and lucrative, global industry. Powerful companies drive research agendas. Seeking constantly to expand their markets, they drive medicalization and disease mongering, selling ordinary human conditions as diseases requiring expensive medical intervention. Conflicts of interest proliferate.

Tragically, too, the clamour for high-tech, death-defying medical fixes and the longing for the magic wand of scientific medicine have led to a terrible neglect of health. It is a truism that prevention is better than cure. We know that

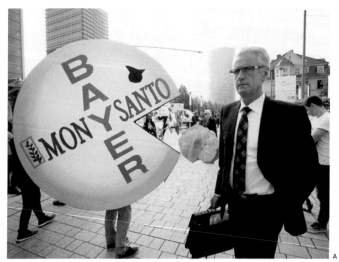

A There is concern that research in medicine, which should be governed by objectivity and scientific neutrality, is increasingly subject to conflicts of interest introduced by powerful commercial players, such as Bayer and Monsanto.

B Medicine is being adapted to lucrative non-therapeutic uses as people seek to improve on ordinary well-being. Seen here is a display of software solutions at a plastic surgery congress in Paris in 2018.

CONCLUSION

A

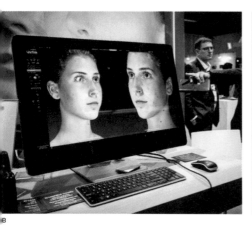

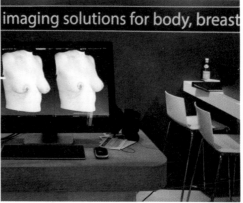

every effect in medicine has a side effect, so where we can we should let our bodies look after themselves, give them a reasonable chance to stay well. But overwhelmingly our energies are poured into expensive cures for disease. Even prevention is being medicalized, with huge sums being spent on medicating the asymptomatic in the hope of deferring future problems. There is no glamour; there are no huge profits in non-medical prevention. We are looking in the wrong direction.

If we draw back from a focus on advanced economies and look globally, the situation is stark. The global spend on malaria research in 2010 was about $547 million. The spend on a cure for HIV/Aids was in the region of $1 billion. According to the International Society of Hair Restoration Surgery, the annual spend on surgical procedures for hair loss is $2 billion. This is not the fault of the medical profession; it is a reflection of unequal economic power and insatiable consumer choice. But it does speak to a dire warping of priorities. Both locally and globally, our health care systems are, if not failing, then buckling terribly.

Change is both necessary and fiercely difficult, but we desperately need to overhaul our health systems.

We must move upstream, get ahead of illness and focus on the ordinary, unglamorous habits of keeping as well as we can. It sounds banal, but yes, we need to eat our greens and move our bodies. Taking on the social forces that make these simple things difficult will not be politically easy, but it needs to be done.

We need to recalibrate our expectations.

We are mortal. We sicken and die. Modern life conspires to veil this truth, but we need to remove the veil. For as long as we deny our embodied frailty, our transience, we will continue to clamour for ever more expensive health care for ever more marginal gains – and still rage indignantly at the world, or our doctors, when the inevitable arrives. It is worth remembering that we have not yet found a cure for the common cold. Perhaps most difficult of all, we need democratically to debate and agree limits to our health care budget. It is plain that we cannot have every health care intervention we want, or even need. The toxic combination of demographic changes, ever-increasing health expectations, co-morbidity, the diseases of affluence, medicalization and the limitless innovations of the medical-industrial complex in search of profits will bankrupt us.

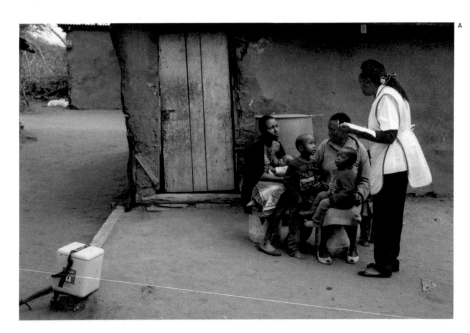

A

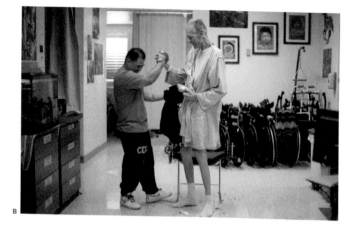

B

Medicine must be understood for what it is: among the most brilliant of our tools.

Justice demands that we strive to distribute it more equally; remediable global inequality in health is a scandal. But we must accept that it will never be the answer to all our ills. On its current trajectory, it threatens to become harmful. Increasingly, our health is in our own hands.

Finally, optimistically, we need to think differently about medicine.

We need to offset our passion for technology and invest in humane, relatively low-tech medical care: the kind of care that is the mainstay of family medicine. Given the shape of the current burden of disease we need a new emphasis: generalism rather than specialization; compassionate care, not all-out war chasing down a cure; a certain acceptance and, ruefully, a certain humility. The belief that we can conquer disease and all but eradicate death may be the most human of fantasies, but that is what it is – a fantasy.

Further Reading

Classical

Galen, *Selected Works* (Oxford: Oxford University Press, 1997)

Harvey, William, *The Circulation of the Blood and Other Writings* (London: Everyman, 1993)

Hippocrates, *Hippocratic Writings* (London: Penguin, 2005)

Vesalius, Andreas, *De Humani Corporis Fabrica (On the Fabric of the Human Body)* (1543)

General

Gawande, Atul, *Being Mortal: Illness, Medicine and What Matters in the End* (London: Profile, 2015)

Gawande, Atul, *Complications: A Surgeon's Notes on an Imperfect Science* (London: Profile, 2010)

Glied, Sherry (Ed), *The Oxford Handbook of Health Economics* (Oxford: Oxford University Press, 2011)

Goldacre, Ben, *Bad Pharma* (London: HarperCollins, 2012)

Goldacre, Ben, *Bad Science* (London: HarperCollins, 2008)

Goldacre, Ben, *I Think You'll Find It's a Bit More Complicated Than That* (London: HarperCollins, 2014)

Healy, David, *Let Them Eat Prozac* (New York: New York University Press, 2004)

Healy, David, *Pharmageddon* (Berkeley: University of California Press, 2012)

Hitchens, Christopher, *Mortality* (London: Atlantic Books, 2012)

Horton, Richard, *Second Opinion: Doctors, Diseases and Decisions in Modern Medicine* (London: Granta, 2003)

Le Fanu, James, *The Rise and Fall of Modern Medicine* (London: Little, Brown, 1999)

Le Fanu, James, *Too Many Pills* (London: Little, Brown, 2018)

Malhotra, Aseem, *A Bitter Pill: A Doctor's Insight into Medical Corruption* (London: Bloomsbury, 2019)

Meier, Barry, *Pain Killer: An Empire of Deceit and the Origin of America's Opioid Epidemic* (New York: Random House, 2018)

Mitford, Jessica, *The American Way of Death Revisited* (London: Virago, 1998)

Moynihan, Ray, *Selling Sickness: How Drug Companies Are Turning Us All into Patients* (Crow's Nest: Allen and Unwin, 2005)

Pickett, Kate, *The Spirit Level: Why More Equal Societies Almost Always Do Better* (London: Bloomsbury, 2009)

Schwarz, Alan, *ADHD Nation: Children, Doctors, Big Pharma, and the Making of an American Epidemic* (New York: Scribner, 2016)

Styron, William, *Darkness Visible* (London: Random House, 2001)

History of Medicine

Bynum, W. F., *The History of Medicine: A Very Short Introduction* (Oxford: Oxford University Press, 2008)

Hollingham, R., *Blood and Guts: A History of Surgery* (London: Random House, 2008)

Longrigg, James, *Greek Medicine from the Homeric to the Heroic Age: A Sourcebook* (New York: Routledge, 1998)

Porter, Roy, *Blood and Guts: A Short History of Medicine* (London: Penguin, 2003)

Porter, Roy, *Madness: A Brief History* (Oxford: Oxford University Press, 2002)

Porter, Roy (Ed), *The Cambridge History of Medicine* (Cambridge: Cambridge University Press, 2006)

Porter, Roy, *The Greatest Benefit to Mankind: A Medical History of Humanity from Antiquity to the Present* (London: HarperCollins, 1997)

Public Health

Berridge, Virginia, *Public Health: A Very Short Introduction* (Oxford: Oxford University Press, 2016)

Marmot, Michael, *The Health Gap* (London: Bloomsbury, 2015)

Spinney, Laura, *Pale Rider: The Spanish Flu of 1918 and How it Changed the World* (London: Random House, 2017)

Sociology of Medicine

Blaxter, Mildred, *Health* (Cambridge: Polity, 2010)

Callahan, Daniel, *Taming the Beloved Beast: How Medical Technology Costs Are Destroying our Health Care System* (Princeton: Princeton University Press, 2009)

Conrad, Peter, *The Medicalization of Society* (Baltimore: The Johns Hopkins University Press, 2007)

Foucault, Michel, *The Birth of the Clinic* (Abingdon: Routledge Classics, 2003)

Illich, Ivan, *Limits to Medicine: Medical Nemesis – The Expropriation of Health* (London: Penguin, 1977)

Nettleton, Sarah, *The Sociology of Health and Illness* (Cambridge: Polity, 2013)

Szasz, Thomas, *The Manufacture of Madness* (New York: Harper and Row, 1970)

Szasz, Thomas, *The Medicalization of Everyday Life* (New York: Syracuse University Press, 2007)

Szasz, Thomas, *The Myth of Mental Illness* (London: HarperCollins, 1984)

Thomas, Carol, *Sociologies of Disability and Illness* (Basingstoke: Palgrave, 2007)

Picture Credits

Every effort has been made to locate and credit copyright holders of the material reproduced in this book. The author and publisher apologize for any omissions or errors, which can be corrected in future editions.

a = above, b = below,
c = centre, l = left, r = right

2 © Paolo Pellegrin / Magnum Photos
4–5 Universal Images Group / Getty Images
6–7 Courtesy Adrian Kantrowitz
8 Javier Larrea / Getty Images
9 Christopher Furlong / Getty Images
10 © Susan Meiselas / Magnum Photos
11 John Moore / Getty Images
12 David Joel / Getty images
13 Jeff Smith / Getty Images
14 Nathan Benn / Corbis via Getty Images
15 Reuters / Faisal Al Nasser
16 Patricia de Melo Moreira / AFP / Getty Images
17 Anthony Kwan / Bloomberg via Getty Images
18–19 Wellcome Collection, London
20 l British Library, London
20 r Wellcome Collection, London
21 British Library, London / Diomedia
22 St. Johns 17 f.7v. St. John's College Library, Oxford
23 British Library, London /

© British Library Board. All Rights Reserved / Bridgeman Images
24 l Wellcome Collection, London
24 r Science Museum, London
25 Epiphanie Medicorum by Ullrich Pinder, 1506
26 Science Museum, London
27 Courtesy Historical Collections & Services, Claude Moore Health Sciences Library, University of Virginia
28 U.S. National Library of Medicine, Bethesda, MD
29 Wellcome Collection, London
30 Private collection. Photo Paul Louis. Courtesy Erasmus House, Brussels
32–33 Wellcome Collection, London
34 Universal Images Group / Christophel Fine Art / Diomedia
35 Florilegius / SSPL / Getty Images
36 The J. Paul Getty Museum, Los Angeles
37 l Jacob A. Riis / Getty Images
37 r Jacob A. Riis / Museum of the City of New York / Getty Images
38 Wellcome Collection, London
39 a Wellcome Collection, London
39 b Hulton-Deutsch Collection / Corbis via Getty Images
40–41 Die Aetiologie der Tuberkulose by Robert Koch. Published by August Hirschwald, Berlin, 1884
42–43 Wellcome Collection, London

44 Roger-Viollet / Topfoto
45 Otis Historical Archives, National Museum of Health and Medicine / Science Photo Library
46 Courtesy Adrian Kantrowitz
47 Courtesy Katrin DeBakey
48 Luca Sage / Getty Images
49 © Burt Glinn / Magnum Photos
50–51 © Peter van Agtmael / Magnum Photos
52 Courtesy Centre for Regenerative Medicine "Stefano Ferrari", University of Modena and Reggio Emilia
53 Joel Prince for The Washington Post via Getty Images
54 l Ontario Pharmacists Association
54 r Meghan McCarthy / The Palm Beach Post via ZUMA Press Inc / Alamy Stock Photo
55 Cory Clark / NurPhoto via Getty Images
56 a Ahikam Seri / Bloomberg via Getty Images
56 b Jasper Juinen / Bloomberg via Getty Images
57 Tom Williams / Getty Images
59 World History Archive / Alamy Stock Photo
60 l DeAgostini / Getty Images
60 r J.L. Kemeny / ISM / Science Photo Library
61 Dr P. Marazzi / Science Photo Library
62 Ruaridh Connellan / Barcroft Images / Barcroft Media via Getty Images
64 BSIP / UIG via Getty Images

Index

References to illustrations
are in **bold**.

addiction 53–5, 78
affluence 15, 66
affordability 14, 88, 99, 107, 134
ageing *see also* life expectancy
  care training **131**
  costs 14, 113–14, 115, 131
  entitlement 112–13
  loneliness 111
  medicalization 62, 78, 88–9,
    113, 131
  quality of life 49
alcohol consumption 111
Aldobrandino of Siena **20**
American Psychiatric
  Association 68
anaesthesia 42
anatomy 27, 28–9, **30**
andropause 92
Annan, Thomas **36**
anthrax 41
anti-ageing treatments **89**
antibiotics 10, 43, 57–9
antidepressants 68, 70–1
anti-psychiatry movement
  67, 68
antipsychotics 45
antiseptics 42, **43**
anti-social behaviour 78
asepsis 42
atherosclerosis 47, 111
attention deficit hyperactivity
  disorder (ADHD) 78, 80–2
attenuated vaccines 40, 41
auscultation 35
austerity 110
autonomy 86
autopsy **28**, 29, 34, 35

baby boomers 112, **113**
back pain 59, 61–2
bacteria 10, **40**–1, 43, 57–9
balance 25
bankruptcy 116, 118, 119, 122
barbers 22, **23**

Barnard, Christiaan 46
Bartisch, Georg **20**
Bazalgette, Jospeh 38, **39**
benzodiazepines 45
Berengario da Carpi, Jacopo **28**
Beveridge, William 15
big data 46
Blaiberg, Philip 46
blindness 102
blood circulation 30, 31
bloodletting **21**, 35
brain **48**
Britain 48, 104, 109, 110, 114,
  120–3
British Psychological Society
  69
Brito, Juan 63
Byrhtferth 22

Callahan, Daniel 115
cancer **49**, 59–60, **61**, 63, 65,
  72, 93
capitalism 98, 99, 133
Cartwright, Samuel 69
CAT (computerized axial
  tomography) scans 44, 45
Chadwick, Edwin 38
Chartran, Théobald **34**
childbirth 11, 78, 79, 83, 116
China **87**, 106
cholera 37, 38, **39**, 41
cholesterol 12
chymoi see humours
classification 31, 32
clinical trials 35, 46, 64, 65, 93
cognitive behaviour therapy 71
common cold 48, 134
co-morbidities 14, 65, 115, 117
compassion 135
complexity 49, 55
conflicts of interest 57, 65, **132**
Conrad, Peter 88, 92, 93
consumer choice 133
contraception 84
Copernicus, Nicolaus 30, 31
cordon sanitaire 39
Corpus Hippocraticum 21, **22**, 23
cosmetic surgery **86**, 87
costs see also affordability
  ageing 113–14, 115, 131

medical-industrial complex
  16, 112
medicalization 88, 99
opportunity costs 108
protests **102**, **104**
rising 123, 127
USA health care 9, 105, **108**,
  109–10, 112, 114, 116–17
cryonics **94**
Cullen, William 32
cupping **20**

Darwin, Erasmus 32
death
  inevitability 95, 96–7, 134,
    135
  as medical failure 11, 72, 95
  medicalization 71–3, 78,
    96–7, 132
  palliative care **11**, **72**, 73,
    94–5, 96
DeBakey, Michael **47**
depression 45, 49, 68, 69–71
diagnosis
  historical development 35
  legitimacy 79
Diagnostic and Statistical
  Manual of Mental Disorders
  (DSM) 68, 69
diagnostics 44, 62, 63
Die Aetiologie der Tuberkulose
  (Koch) **40**
disease *see also* medicalization;
  morbidities
  diagnostic thresholds
    62, 64, 69
  early beliefs 22–4
  emergent infections
    84, **85**
  endemic 33
  epidemic 33
  germ theory 31, 38,
    41–2, 43
  lifestyle 10, 15, 47–8,
    66, 111
  miasmatic theory 38
  ontologically separate
    31–2
  as spectrum 84–5
  disease mongering **86**, 87, **132**

dissection 27, 28–9, **30**
distributive justice 122
DNA 46, 49, 68
DNA sequencing 62, 63
Doctors Without Borders **126**
drug overdoses 53–4
drugs *see* pharmaceuticals
Drugs for Neglected Diseases
    Initiative 126, 127
Duane Reade **77**

Ebola **85**
economic ultra-liberalism 104,
    105
elective surgery 104
electro-convulsive therapy **45**
embolisms 64, 65
empiricism 22, 23, 27, 28, 29
endemic disease 33
end of life care **11**, 73, 94–5,
    96, 130
entitlement 112, **113**
environment 15, 36, 49
environmental degradation 107
epidemic disease 33
epigenetics 48, 49
Epiphanie Medicorum (Pinder)
    25
equality of access 88, 103, 104,
    105, 106–7, 117–19, 121–2,
    124–6, 135
erectile dysfunction 90–1
ethics 49, 82–3, 85–6
evolution 58
examination 35
exercise **14, 67, 110,** 134
expectations 16, 56, 71, 98, 104,
    112, **113**, 134

On the Fabric of the Human Body
    (Vesalius) **29**
false positives 65
family history 22
fentanyl 54
filoviruses 84, 85
Fleming, Alexander 43
Florey, Howard 43
food 15, **66, 117,** 125, 134
Foucault, Michel 67
France 33, 34, **35, 42**

Gadsden, Henry 98
Galen of Pergamum 26, 27, 29
generalization 135
genetic engineering 14, 52–3
genetic therapies 102
Gensen, Kanda **32**
germ theory 31, 41–2, 43
grief 85, 86
gross domestic product (GDP)
    104, 105
*Guild Book of the Barber
    Surgeons of York* **23**

hair loss 133
Halappanavar, Savita **84**
Harvey, William 30, 31
Hawking, Stephen 121, 122
healers, traditional 27
health care
    affordability 14, 88, 99,
        102–3, 107, 134
    equality of access 88, 103,
        104, 105, 106–7, 117–19,
        121–2, 124–6, 135
    as global business 16, **17**
    global expenditure
        comparisons 105, 106,
        107, **108,** 109–10, 114,
        117, 133
    humane 135
    payment models 103–4,
        121
heart 30, **31,** 46
heart disease 111
heredity 49
Hippocrates 20, 21, 22, 24
history
    19th century 34–42
    20th century 43–4, 131
    ancient Greeks 20, 21, 22,
        24, 26, 27
    Enlightenment 30–3
    Japan **32**
    medieval **20,** 21, 22–4, 27
    Renaissance **20, 24–5,**
        28–30
    Romans 27
Hoffmann-La Roche 45
holistic medicine 22, 23
homeostasis 25

hormone replacement therapy
    (HRT) 92–3
hospices 96, 130
hospitals 33, **34,** 35, **107**
humours **22,** 23–4
Huntington's chorea 14, 15
hygiene **9,** 42
hyper-individualism 99

iatrogenic illness 9, 120
Illich, Ivan 78, 86
illness *see* disease
immortality 47, 95
immune suppression 46, 47
India 103, 106, 107
individualism 99, 105, 114, 115
infections, nosocomial 9
innovation 112
inoculation 33, 40
insurance 79, 103, 105, 116, 118
intelligence 82, 83
intensive care units **96,** 97, 116
interventions 64, **134**
Ioannidis, John 65
ischaemic heart disease 111, 114

Japan 110, **111**
justice 16

Koch, Robert 40, 41

Labiaplasty 86, 87
Laënnec, René **34**
Laing, RD 67
Lawson, Nigel 120
LDL cholesterol 12
Le Fanu, James 113
legitimacy 79, 85
lesions 34
liberal individualism 114, 115
life expectancy *see also*
    mortality
        19th century urbanization
        37
        co-morbidities 49
        decrease 110
        global comparisons 110,
        124–5
        health care expenditure
        109–11

immortality 47
increase 14, 71, **73**, 131
opioid dependency 10,
53–4, 110
USA health care 117, 119
Lifeline Express **107**
lifestyle diseases 10, 15, 47–8,
66, 111
lifestyle drugs 80, 82, 90–1
Li Livres dou Santé
(Aldobrandino) 20
Linnaeus 32
Lister, Joseph 42, **43**
lithium 45, 68
London's 'great stink' 38, **39**
loneliness 111
longevity *see* life expectancy
Louis, Pierre 35
Lower, Richard **31**
Luxturna 102

magic 22, **26**
malaria 33
malnutrition 66, 67
mammography **64**, 65
Marcus Aurelius 26
market failure 59, 125, 126
Marmot, Michael 117
masculinity 88, 90, 92
May, Theresa **122**
medical imperialism 90
medical-industrial complex 16,
17, 112, 124
medicalization 11, 12, 13, 67,
76–9, 81, 83–94, 96–9, 113,
131–2
The Medicalization of Society
(Conrad) 88
Medical Nemesis (Illich) 78
medical triad 24–5, 36
menopause 92–3
mental health
20th century development
44–5
ADHD 78, 80–2
diagnostic thresholds 69
genetics 49
legitimacy 79
medicalization 13, 67, 78
psychiatry 66–7

social norms 68–9
Merck 98
miasmatic theory 38
microbiology 40
micronutrient malnutrition 66,
67
military health **44**
Modafinil 82
Mondino de' Luzzi 29
Montaigne, Michel de 89
moral hazard 122, 123
morbidities
affluence 15, 66
ageing 49
co-morbidities 14, 65, 115,
117
side effects 56, 60
Moreton, Samuel G. **32**
morgues 34, **35**
mortality *see also* life
expectancy
child **36**, 37, 71
clinical trials 93
inevitability 95, 96–7,
134, 135
infant 11, 37, 71, 83–4, 117,
119, 124–5
maternal 11, 83–4, 125
over-diagnosis 63
surgical 42–3
*On the Motion of the Heart and
Blood* (Harvey) 31
Moynihan, Ray 64
MRI scans 61, **81**
MRSA 58, 59
Mundinus 29

Naloxone **54**, 55
National Health Service (NHS)
48, 104, 114, 120–3
natural laws 22
On the Nature of Man
(attr. Polybus) 23
neglected tropical diseases
(NTDs) 126, 127
neuroscience 46, 47, **48**, 68
neurotransmitters 68
Newton, Isaac 30
nosocomial infections 9
nosologies 32

Obamacare 56, 104, **105**
obesity 14, 15, 66, 111, 117
obesogenic environment 15
oestrogen 92, 93
Olympics 82, **83**
ontologically separate 31–2
Ophthalmodouleia (Bartisch) **20**
opioids 10, 52, 53–4, **55**, 56, 110
opportunity costs 108
organ transplants 46
osteoporosis **92**
over-diagnosis 62, 63
over-treatment 60, 63, 65
OxyContin 54

pain
anaesthesia 42
back pain 59, 61–2
benefits 86
early beliefs 23
painkillers 54–5 *see also*
opioids
palliative care 52, **72**, 73, 94–5,
96, 130
palpation 35
Paracelsus 30
parasites 124
Paris 33, 34, **35**, **42**
Pasteur, Louis 40, 41
pathology 34–5, 36
patient-doctor relationship
34, 36
patient groups 79, 92, **93**
patients
expectations 16, 56, 71, 98,
104, 112, **113**, 134
justice 16
trust 17
penicillin 43
percussion 35
performance enhancement 82,
83, 90–1
Pfizer 90, 91
pharmaceuticals *see also* side
effects
Drugs for Neglected
Diseases Initiative 126
enhancement drugs 82
global distribution
inequalities 124, **126**

manufacture 12–13, 56, 130
market failure 59
mental health 45
profit 16, 57, 98–9, 126, 127, 132, 133
Pickett, Kate 117
Pinder, Ullrich 25
placebos 64, 70, 93
plastic surgery 87
politics 56, 57, 122, 123 see also state intervention
Polybus 23
polypharmacy 14, 15, 113, 115
population screening 60, 61, 64–5
Porter, Roy 21
post-mortems see autopsy
poverty 33, 36, 37–8, 55, 105, 107, 116, 119, 125
prenatal care 10, 116
prescriptions
    conflicts of interest 57
    opioid dependency 53–4, 55, 56
prevention 12, 132–4
primal therapy 70
primary care 120, 121
privacy 86, 87
privatization 121
profit 16, 17, 57, 98–9, 126, 127, 132, 133
progestin 93
prostate cancer 59–60, 61
protests 102, 104, 121, 126
psychiatry 66–71
psychogenic ailments 90, 91
psychotherapy 70
public health 36–40, 114, 114, 115

quality of life 11, 49, 93
quinine 33

rabies 41
randomized controlled trials (RCTs) 64, 65
rationing 123
religion 22, 26
Report on the Sanitary Condition of the Labouring Population

of Great Britain (Chadwick) 38
reproductive choice 84
research funding 64, 65
On the Revolutions of the Heavenly Spheres (Copernicus) 30, 31
Riis, Jacob A. 37
risk avoidance 95
risk factors 9, 62, 125
Ritalin (methylphenidate) 80, 81, 82
robots, surgical 8
Rontgen, William 44
Rosenthal, Jared 62

Sams, William 35
sanitation 38, 39, 106
schistosomiasis 124, 126
scientific revolution 30
screening see population screening
selective serotonin reuptake inhibitors (SSRIs) 68
serotonin 68, 71
sewers 38, 39
sexual potency 90–1
Shakespeare, William 88
side effects 12, 55, 56, 60, 80, 85–6, 95, 113, 133 see also risk factors
Sinconis, Jen 116
skin grafts 52–3
Snow, John 38
social control 67
social health insurance (SHI) 103
social media 86, 87
social pressure 87
social support 79
Sophie's Choice (Styron) 69
Spark Therapeutics 102
specialization 17, 25, 135
The Spirit Level (Pickett & Wilkinson) 117
sport 82, 83
staphylococci 43
state intervention 39–40, 67, 114, 115 see also politics
statins 12
statistics 35, 65, 114, 124–5

St Cosmas 24
stem cells 52
stigma 79, 85
Styron, William 69–70
surgery
    19th century development 42–3
    20th century development 46
    elective 104
    modern progress 130
    on trains 107
Szasz, Thomas 67

Taming the Beloved Beast (Callahan) 115
taxation 104
testosterone 92
thyroid cancer 63
Tractatus de Corde (Lower) 31
trust 17
tuberculosis 32, 33, 40, 41, 58, 59

uncertainty 59, 60, 62
urbanization 33, 36, 37, 106, 107
urine 24, 25
USA health care 9, 105, 108, 109–10, 112, 114, 116–20, 122

vaccination 40, 41, 44, 134 see also inoculation
Valium 45
Vesalius, Andreas 29
Viagra 90–1
Voltaire 21
votive offerings 26

waiting lists 123
Washkansky, Louis 46
water sanitation 38, 39, 106
well-being 13, 77, 98, 134
Western medicine
    hegemony 8
    progress 9
Wilkinson, Richard 117
World Health Organization (WHO) 66, 83

X-rays 44

Acknowledgments:
The author would like to thank his old
friend Matthew Taylor for sparking the
idea, and for more intellectual stimulation
and companionship than I can properly
acknowledge. Thanks also to Becky Gee
and Jane Laing, my kind and undemanding
editors, and to Phoebe Lindsley and Tristan
de Lancey for their thoughtful and provocative
picture edit and design. And finally to Imelda
and my boys Finlay and Dominic for
their endless patience and good humour.

First published in the United Kingdom in 2019
by Thames & Hudson Ltd, 181A High Holborn,
London WC1V 7QX

Is Medicine Still Good For Us? © 2019
Thames & Hudson Ltd, London

General Editor: Matthew Taylor
Text by Julian Sheather

For image copyright information, see pp. 138–139

British Library Cataloguing-in-Publication Data
A catalogue record for this book is available from
the British Library

ISBN 978-0-500-29458-1

Printed and bound in Slovenia by
DZS-Grafik d.o.o.

To find out about all our publications,
please visit **www.thamesandhudson.com**.
There you can subscribe to our e-newsletter,
browse or download our current catalogue,
and buy any titles that are in print.